WEEDY WISDOM

for the Curious Forager

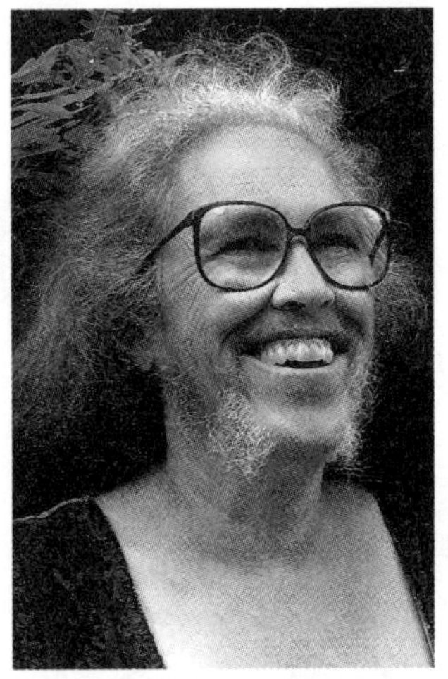

© Anne E. Stone

About the Author

Rebecca Randall Gilbert discovered her love of foraging at age six when she spent the summer with her grandmother on Martha's Vineyard. She has been exploring the subject—and grazing on the same farm—ever since. She teaches a variety of rural skills at Native Earth Teaching Farm, which she and her husband opened to the public in 2002.

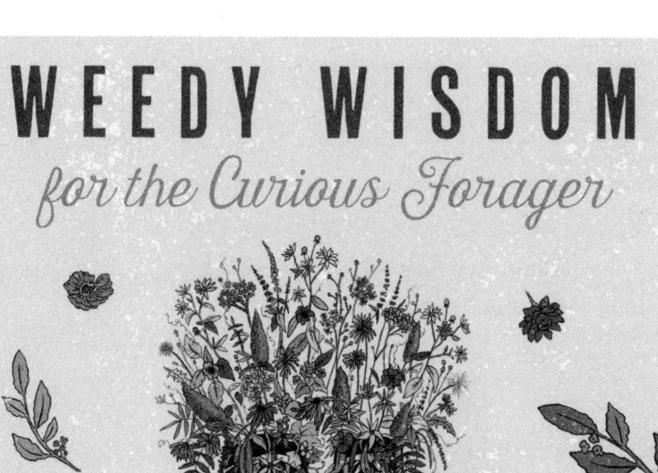

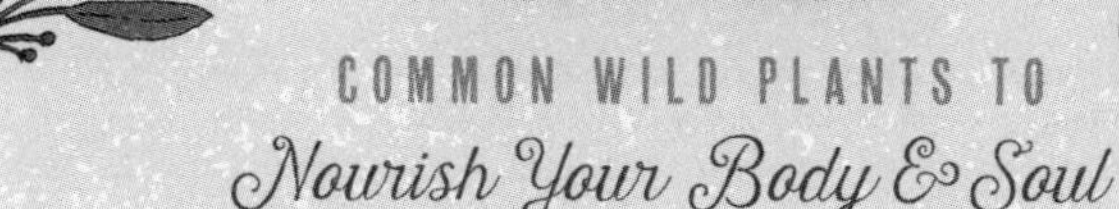

REBECCA RANDALL GILBERT

Llewellyn Publications
Woodbury, Minnesota

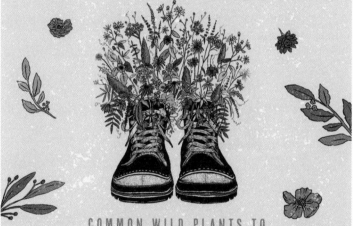

First Edition
First Printing, 2022

Book design by Colleen McLaren
Cover art and interior art by Kaari Selvin
Cover design by Kevin R. Brown
Photo on page xxv by Kelsey Cosby

Library of Congress Cataloging-in-Publication Data
Names: Gilbert, Rebecca Randall, author.
Title: Weedy wisdom for the curious forager : common wild plants to nourish your body & soul / Rebecca Randall Gilbert.
Description: First edition. | Woodbuy, Minnesota : Llewellyn Publications, [2022] | Includes index.
Identifiers: LCCN 2022001899 (print) | LCCN 2022001900 (ebook) | ISBN 9780738772073 (paperback) | ISBN 9780738772158 (ebook)
Subjects: LCSH: Wild plants, Edible—East (U.S.)—Identification. | Wild foods—East (U.S.) | Cooking (Wild foods)—East (U.S.) | Medicinal plants—East (U.S.) | Materia medica, Vegetable—East (U.S.)
Classification: LCC QK98.5.U6 G55 2022 (print) | LCC QK98.5.U6 (ebook) | DDC 581.6/32—dc23/eng/20220307
LC record available at https://lccn.loc.gov/2022001899
LC ebook record available at https://lccn.loc.gov/2022001900

Llewellyn Publications
A Division of Llewellyn Worldwide Ltd.
2143 Wooddale Drive
Woodbury, MN 55125-2989
www.llewellyn.com
Printed in the United States of America

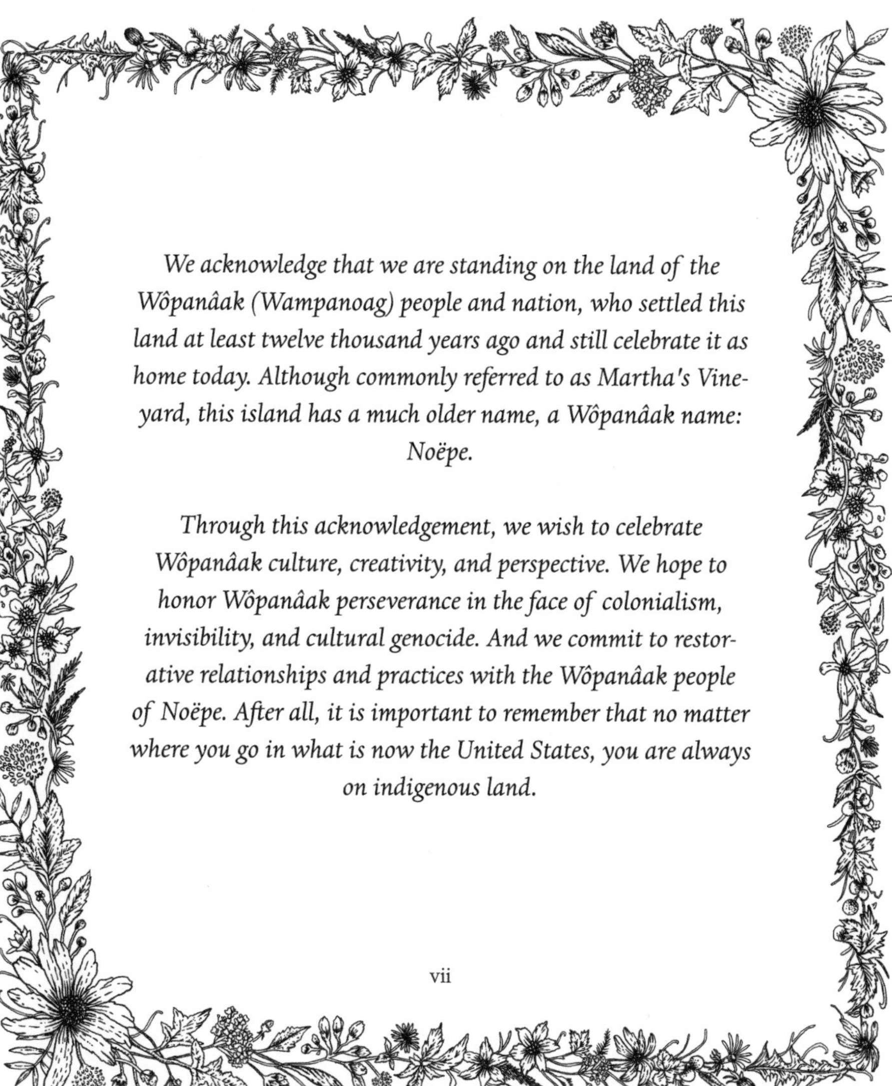

We acknowledge that we are standing on the land of the Wôpanâak (Wampanoag) people and nation, who settled this land at least twelve thousand years ago and still celebrate it as home today. Although commonly referred to as Martha's Vineyard, this island has a much older name, a Wôpanâak name: Noëpe.

Through this acknowledgement, we wish to celebrate Wôpanâak culture, creativity, and perspective. We hope to honor Wôpanâak perseverance in the face of colonialism, invisibility, and cultural genocide. And we commit to restorative relationships and practices with the Wôpanâak people of Noëpe. After all, it is important to remember that no matter where you go in what is now the United States, you are always on indigenous land.

Contents

Plant Portraits

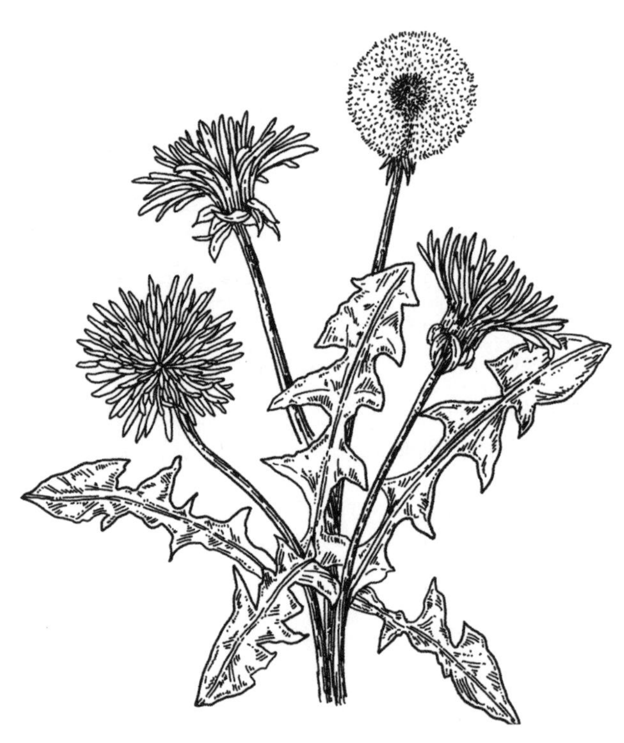

Recipes

BEVERAGES

Crafts

Practices

List of Helpful Lists

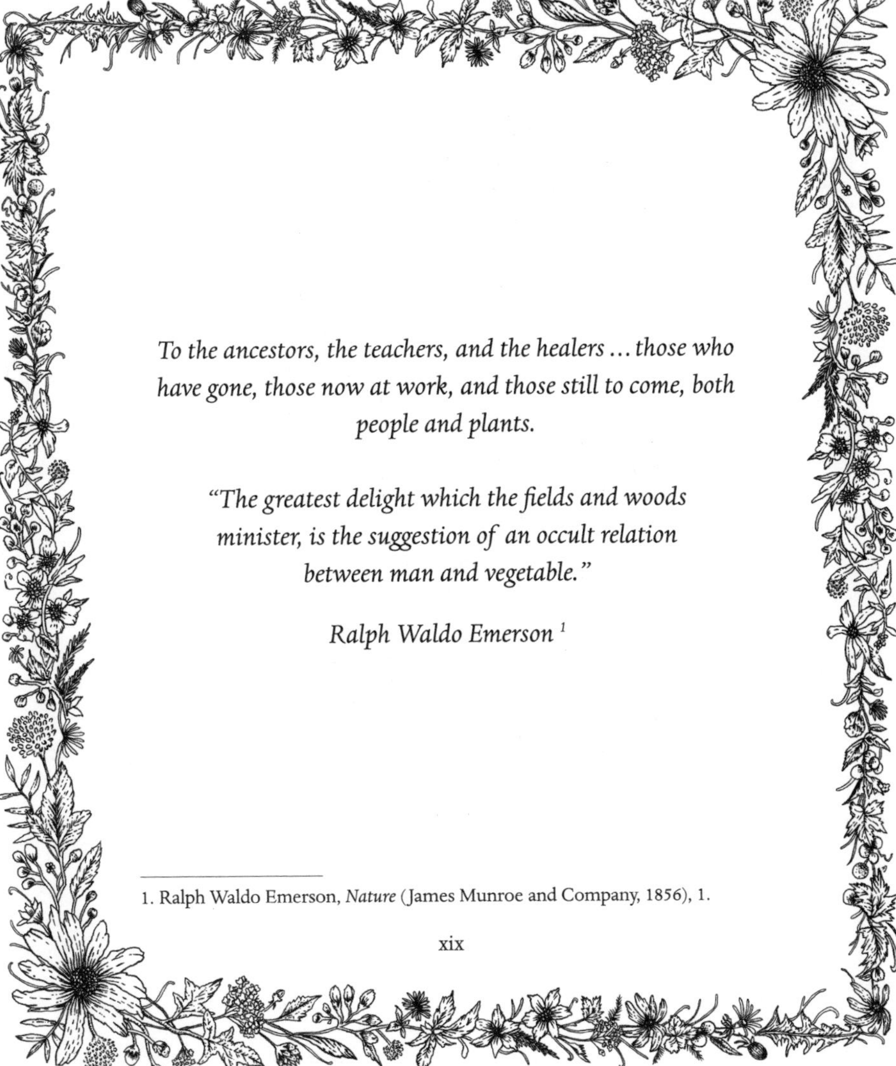

To the ancestors, the teachers, and the healers ... those who have gone, those now at work, and those still to come, both people and plants.

"The greatest delight which the fields and woods minister, is the suggestion of an occult relation between man and vegetable."

Ralph Waldo Emerson [1]

1. Ralph Waldo Emerson, *Nature* (James Munroe and Company, 1856), 1.

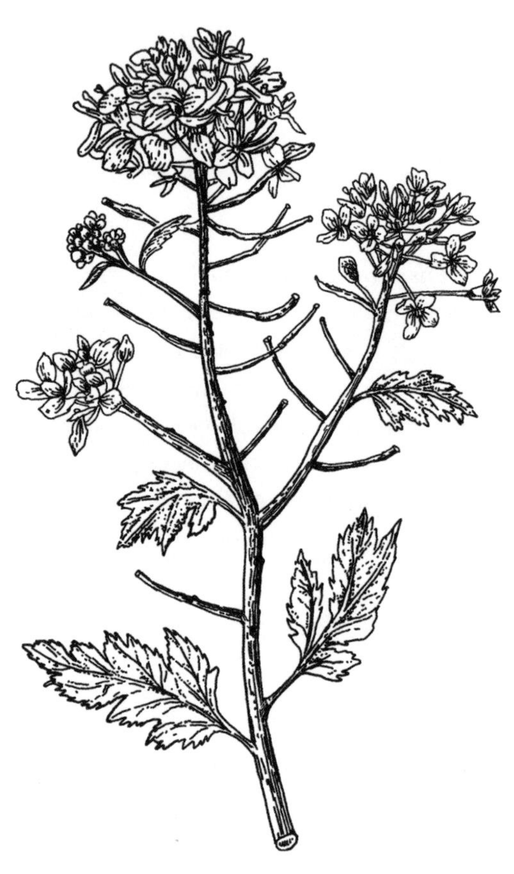

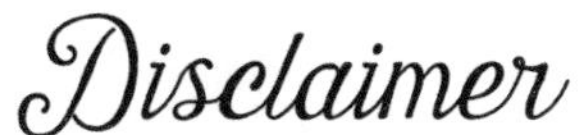

Disclaimer

We make no claims for cures or medical treatments; discuss these with your most trusted healthcare professionals. The purpose of foraging, and the subject of this book, is primarily the provision of food. In general, flavor is tied to a rich and wholesome nutritional composition, and consuming delicious food is good for people. So is getting outside and paying attention to nature, and so is having fun. I personally have benefited from foraging both physically and mentally, and have shared details here as examples, but your situation will be different, and, like mine, will require your personal evaluations and decisions. I wish you good health and good eating.

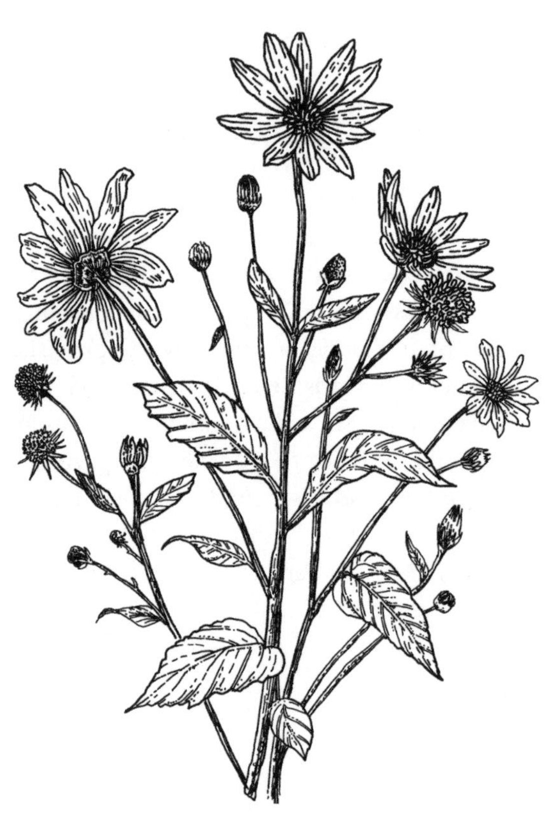

Preface

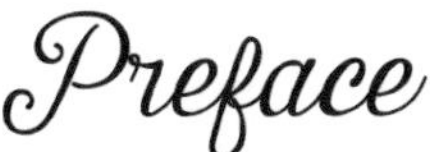

This book arose from a season of foraging and conversation that took place as a collaboration between Native Earth Teaching Farm and Camp Jabberwocky on the island of Martha's Vineyard. The dynamic that evolved from this collaboration informed the vivid and accessible knowledge in this book, so it might be helpful to begin by introducing the participants.

About Native Earth Teaching Farm

Native Earth Teaching Farm is located on a glacial moraine on a watershed between the north and south shores of Martha's Vineyard, Wampanoag land. The farm opened to the public in 2002 to share its healing and educational powers with a wider audience. There, Rebecca Randall Gilbert and her husband raise animals and plants to their heart's content, and Rebecca teaches rural skills and fiber arts to anyone who shows an interest, from toddlers to elders. From community gardens to goat school to bubbling dye pots to herbal potions, there's always some sort of experiment or investigation going on, or some kind of project taking root. Famous for their compost, the friendliness of their goats, their delicious local food, and their ornery, old-fashioned ways, these farmers are doing their best to carry forward the skills and joys of the past into a new and different future. Volunteers and coconspirators are always welcome to contact Rebecca and plot an adventure.

Camp Jabberwocky

Camp Jabberwocky is the oldest sleepaway camp for people with disabilities in America. It was founded in the early 1950s by Helen "Hellcat" Lamb. Jabberwocky all started with one woman's desire to improve the lives of people in our communities. Helen Lamb was taking a short vacation from her job as a speech pathologist and was feeling a little guilty that she was there on Martha's Vineyard sitting on the beach with her own three children, while the children she worked with were left behind in the hot city, under bad conditions, with no vacation in view and no break for the parents … out of this single moment came the prospect of Camp Jabberwocky. For over sixty-five years, Camp Jabberwocky has been going strong with Hellcat's mission to provide campers with a phenomenal experience full of adventure, friendship, and challenge. Hellcat was a force. She had a simple saying that lives on to this very day: "There is a way; find it."

To Hellcat, accessibility didn't matter; if there was an activity to do or an adventure to endure, camp did it. She had this can-do attitude that made Jabberwocky happen.

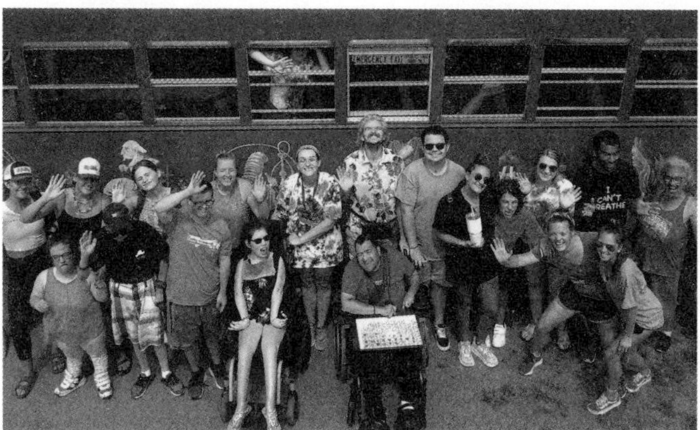

© Kelsey Cosby

The Collaboration That Led to This Book

When the farm and the camp found one another, it was a happy match, because all concerned like to have fun while never avoiding the most difficult subjects. The project that spawned this book was a series of foraging classes, and the wide-ranging discussions that developed during and after class. Here, the curious reader will find a guide to the specifics of plant communication and some homegrown philosophy to help establish a deeper understanding of the fluid and interactive relationships between people and plants. This theoretical groundwork finds practical expression in the following chapters, each based on a class with Camp Jabberwocky held at the farm, and each covering a different aspect of foraging.

Foreword

BY MICHAEL LEON

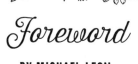

It was a balmy June morning when Camp Jabberwocky arrived at the Native Earth Teaching Farm. We poured out of our red bus and raced for the goats. "What's this one's name, what's that one's name? How old are they, which one's the momma goat?" We were splayed out over a bed of hay, laughing and yipping as the goats climbed over our laps and licked our faces. With great effort, we eventually pried ourselves away from the goats and slowly made our way back to the bus (it was almost lunch time, after all). A few of us lingered around the farm, curiously eyeing the plants and flowers that surrounded us.

"Do you have any medicinal plants in your garden?" my friend Scott asked.

"Honestly," Rebecca leaned in close to Scott's wheelchair as if readying to share a secret. "I like to use the weeds."

"The weeds?!" I said, louder than intended, almost sure she was joking. *But weeds aren't good for anything*, I thought to myself.

"Weeds take what they want, so they're very rich in nutrients. And over the years, I've found that if I pay attention to what weeds are growing around the farm, they seem to anticipate what I might need during the year."

To say my curiosity was piqued would be an understatement. Rebecca was describing a world full of rich magic and wonder that lay right beneath our feet. There was a simplicity and deep knowing in her words that made the weeds feel like sacred allies waiting to be awakened, waiting to be invited to the table. Some knowledge is gained through years of hard work and experience, but there is another kind that feels uniquely preternatural. And the sympathy and understanding with which Rebecca's related to the earth felt immediately and especially gifted.

I was fascinated—both with Rebecca and with the wild, magical world of weeds she spoke of. And I wasn't the only one! As the weeks went by and we continued to visit Native Earth, Jabberwocky's collective attention gradually shifted from playing with the goats to asking questions about the newest weeds in Rebecca's yard.

And so, our foraging class was born—a collaboration between Jabberwocky and Native Earth, inspired by Rebecca's rare passion and our unquenchable curiosity. The next summer, we returned every week for classes to learn (and eat!) our way through the native plants of Martha's Vineyard.

I trust you'll find this book to be, like its author, full of wisdom and magic. Let these pages be your invitation to the delicious and unexpected world of secret greens—hiding in plain sight, and just waiting to be tasted.

Let the foraging begin!

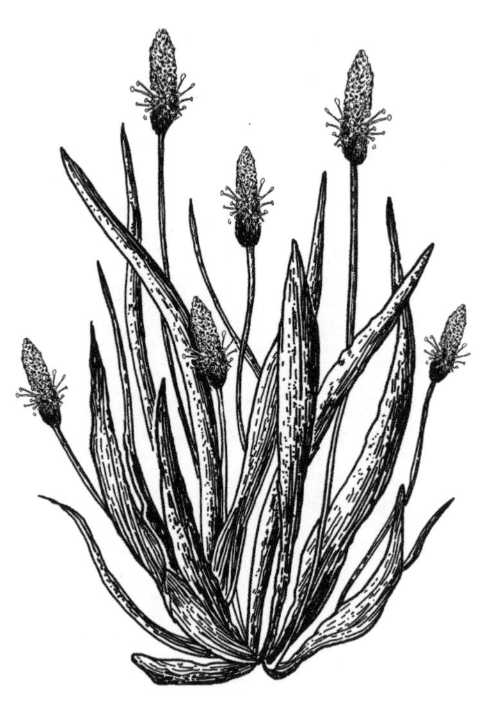

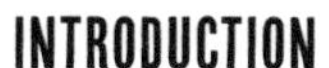

INTRODUCTION

Breathing with Plants

This book is for anyone who has, or would like to have, an affinity for plants. Based on a series of foraging classes for complete beginners, it starts with a discussion of comfort and safety, and goes on to cover methods and techniques that anyone can use to amplify and enrich their connections and conversations with the plants around them. After that, we'll get into specific plants, preparations, and recipes.

First, though, let's take time to appreciate the intimate relationship that already exists between ourselves and the plants of the world, past and present. Children learn in school that plants breathe in carbon dioxide and breathe out oxygen, while animals like us do the reverse. The plant kingdom, their ancestors the fungi, and the even older cyanobacteria had already oxygenated the earth's atmosphere long before animals came on the scene. That's one reason I consider plants to be our wise elders, even the little sprouts. For each of us personally, our individual relationship with the world's plants began at birth, when we took our first gasping breath of oxygen-rich air … and this relationship continues with each breath we take.

Many traditions of meditation and methods for the cultivation of inner wisdom ask us to focus attention on the breath. This simple practice has profound benefits. It connects people to plants, and also to the interfaces between one's physical interior and the outside world as well as to those between body and mind. Breathing operates at the border of consciousness. Usually, when we don't think about it, it happens automatically. When we bring awareness to breathing, we can intentionally increase fire, activity, and adrenaline by entering a fight-or-flight mode through fast, shallow panting, or we may choose to engage the calming, restorative influence of the parasympathetic nervous system by taking slower, deeper breaths. Checking in with the breath can help us understand how we are feeling, and shifting the breath can influence the body's response. Because it is always changing, attention to the breath requires our presence in the always-transitional moving target of the current moment. This makes attention to breath particularly useful when working with difficult entrenched emotions and traumatic memories, as healing ourselves and the world often requires.

Because we humans have developed a problematic relationship with the rest of nature, we have some justification in thinking of ourselves as toxic and dangerous. When we are engaged in behavior that leads to pollution, exploitation, and the disruption of natural systems of balance, this view is correct. More than mere preludes to action, words, thoughts, and beliefs can also be toxic. In fact, early research into talking to plants helped give momentum to the idea that negative self-talk, especially as taught to children, has damaging effects far beyond hurt feelings in the moment. A plant that is verbally abused on a regular basis becomes stunted and weakened. The same plant, under the same physical care, will begin to thrive when addressed kindly. It is very sad that many of us are prone to critical and negative rants and harmful thoughts directed within. Talking to the plants around us can redirect unhealthy inner chatter into more realistic and wholesome channels. Like talking to pets, wild birds, the departed, and so on, this practice widens awareness to include other beings, promotes recognition of our place in a complex web of ecosystems, and reduces the focus on the self. The resulting natural awareness and appreciation of the world around us tends to make us less drawn to toxic behavior and negativity in general.

In any case, when we breathe with plants, the "stale" or "depleted" or "bad" air we exhale is *not* another way that we dump our garbage. True, it clears and cleans our lungs and blood, allowing us a regular and repeated opportunity for releasing everything that we no longer need, but it is far from toxic. Instead, it is a pure and direct gift to those who have nurtured and fed us all along—the oxygen-producing plants. In fact, gently blowing an outbreath onto a plant is like giving oxygen to a person—it's an energizing breath of extra-fresh air.

Whenever your mind is full, or if you find yourself out of your depth, feel free to return to the simple practice of breathing with plants. This close, constant, mutually beneficial connection is always available. We don't need to pay attention, or to know or name the plants from which our oxygen comes or to whom our carbon dioxide flows. The relationship sustains us all nevertheless. Based on this ample and secure foundation, this exchange of gifts, we are well positioned to explore and expand our involvement with the weeds around us, seeking to discover additional nourishing connections between ourselves and common plants.

Plant Communication: A Manual

I have sometimes called myself a weed witch, because wild plants are some of my best friends and most profound teachers in life. It is the ways they (and the ecosystems and cyclic patterns of which they form a part) have taught and healed and helped me that I have attempted to communicate here. "Talking to plants" sounds esoteric and even impossible to many people, but we all eat, so it is through the taste buds and the need for nourishment that I try to make the connections between people of any experience level and the energetic magic of vivid, friendly, available local plants. It's not necessary to "believe" in magic to forage, but I emphasize the real, easily discernable magic that is already there whenever we connect in this way, so that we all become more comfortable with acknowledging and using intuition and plant consciousness in our own spiritual healing journeys as well as in the field, the kitchen, and at the table.

How to Begin

Once you've taken a deep breath, exactly how does one go about learning to communicate with plants? Most people new to foraging initially worry that they will make a mistake and poison themselves or others, and while relatively rare, this sort of mistake has indeed happened. So, let's begin by talking about safety for beginning foragers. It's easy to say DO NOT EAT ANYTHING YOU DON'T RECOGNIZE. But how do we learn to recognize? At first, everything seems like a "sea of green." You will not be a safe forager until you have passed this stage and can pick out distinguishing details of plants and their environments. This is not difficult, but it takes time. Be patient—the complex skills you are developing have lifelong benefits.

Imagine that you have moved into a new neighborhood. At first, everyone is a stranger. After a while, you've met a few people, and there are others you recognize. You may not know their names or what they do, but you've seen them around. Bit by bit, you learn things about them. When you've lived in the neighborhood long enough, you'll notice any new elements or unusual behavior right away. Developing this kind of systemic familiarity cannot be rushed.

I invite you to hang out in the neighborhood of wild plants. Get to know those you see frequently. If you're a beginner, start with one you really like—the more common, the better. Since our eventual goal as foragers is nourishing and delicious food in abundance, there isn't much point in targeting rare species that are struggling in your region. Start with those that "stick out," or "call to you," or "get in your face"—the friendly ones: the weeds.

Long before you are ready to harvest for food, you can get to know some friendly weeds. Here are some specific techniques that can really speed up the process.

- **VISUAL ARTS:** Using whatever mediums you prefer, portray all or part of your chosen plant. Your aim is not the finished artwork, but the noticing, so you can suspend judgment and simply play, explore, and actively observe.
- **MUSIC AND PERFORMANCE:** Song, dance, and poetry recitation are traditional offerings to plants in many cultures, times, and places.

Don't steal or borrow—develop your own. Those that arise spontaneously are the most effective.

- **HIDE AND SEEK:** Pause now and then, here and there. Can you see your plant? Touch it? How far would you have to go to find it? When you see your plant, wink, or wave, and say hello in your mind. Or you may say, "Tag, you're it!"
- **INTIMACY:** We learn a lot about one another in close quarters. Put a sprig or branch in a vase where you will see it often. Admire it frequently and compost the remains with respect, perhaps returning them to the soil around the source plant, with thanks.
- **PERSISTENCE:** Follow your plant through its cycles of life and death. Learn the way it first sprouts from the soil, and when. Notice how it behaves right before flowering, the shape and feel of its seeds, and the way the dead stalks hold clinging snow. Many people recommend getting to know a plant for a year or more before beginning to use it in any way.
- **CULTURE:** Unless it's invasive, propagate your plant. Study the conditions under which it grows best, and start to notice places where it would be happy. Try growing it as a houseplant. Collect and share seeds. Seed dispersal is a benefit that we animals have offered to plants since time immemorial, allowing them to enjoy our animated mobile tendencies.
- **RESEARCH:** Ask yourself some riddles. You may find yourself wondering about something that can be tested. Make your best guess

first, and then observe until you have satisfied your curiosity. Plants and situations change, so direct observation in the field is more valuable than secondary information from books or past observations. Since plants express themselves slowly over time, you may want to keep records.

Keep in mind that plants are much older than animals, and the allies of the plants, bacteria and fungi, are more ancient still. They are our elders and ancestors, and it behooves us to act accordingly. Just as with our human elders, try not to be impetuous. Be respectful and listen before talking. Learn what to avoid, and don't mess with strangers. Always say thank you, and lend a hand where you see a need. Greet them, touch them, bring small gifts. Be completely honest with them at all times. Turn to your elders, the weeds, when you need help and healing. Ask them directly for their assistance. The depth of their wisdom and generosity never fails to amaze me.

Unfriendly Weeds

There are some plants that will make you sick, or give you a rash, and some can kill you. You will feel more confident once you know the ones to avoid. Wait until you are certain of what something is before using it.

As long as you don't eat them by mistake, most plants won't bother you. The exceptions are those that can irritate your skin as you pass through them. Poison ivy is very common in our region, and poison sumac, though fairly rare, can cause a painful rash. Several other species may cause skin reactions in sensitive individuals.

Plants vary by species, by location, and by individual. Poison ivy, for example, is extremely variable. It can look quite different from place to place—sometimes a ground cover, sometimes a climbing vine, with a lot of variation in leaf types. It can be very confusing to identify. In such cases, it's helpful to look for those attributes that are always present—the plant's signature. With poison ivy, there are "leaves of three," striking fall color, and the way little clinging rootlets grow off the side of the stem like caterpillar feet. This last attribute can be seen even in the root, and at all seasons of the year. Learn to recognize these plants in all their forms, and you will find that they become friendlier and easier to avoid. They can be great teachers in the art of noticing. Meanwhile, it is always a good idea to approach a completely new plant with caution and respect. One of the functions of such plants is to keep us careful, respectful, and paying attention. If any doubt remains, more time and study are required.

Fungi are outside the scope of this work, a kingdom unto themselves, with their own cryptic languages. They are even more ancient and mysterious and magical than plants, and harder to get to know. However, the techniques outlined here may also be helpful in gaining greater familiarity with fungi.

Green Literacy: Learning from Plants

Becoming familiar enough with a plant to safely and accurately identify it under any conditions is a necessary first step in developing your relationship. You and this plant have become like acquaintances ... people who call each other by name and exchange pleasantries. You would recognize such a person even if they dyed their hair or changed jobs. You could say that you know them. However, when true friendships develop, they can go much deeper. The depth of communication and potential healing that is possible from such relationships goes far beyond easy familiarity. It becomes simple and natural to share information and revelation in ways that boggle the rational mind, and to understand one another intuitively the way lovers, siblings, or longtime friends sometimes do.

For these kinds of deep, mutually beneficial friendships to develop, we need language. Part of what is required is the ability to hear and trust intuition, a skill that ripens with practice, testing, and play. This provides the listening heart that is one half of communication. What about the other half, the vocabulary of plant speech? This is something that each person develops in the course of their relationships with plants and with nature in general. The more you know, and the more different types of knowing that you are able to bring to bear on a situation, the more avenues lie open for connection and communication to take place.

Modern science focuses on aspects of plant biology that can be measured and replicated by different people in any time and place. Aspects that can be considered relatively objective and permanent include Latin name and family, looks (phenotype), active constituents, chemical makeup, genetic structure, and so on. These more stable attributes are necessary to focus on when you are first learning to identify plants, but they amount to the plant sitting there, not saying anything... playing dead. If you want conversation, you have to go beyond the fixed and enter into the fluid, flexible, and fleeting.

Traditional herbalists who "talk" with nature generally have many more perspectives on a plant than are acceptable under the scientific worldview. Subjectivity, not objectivity, is the goal. We consider as valid input much that would not be eligible as evidence to a modern scientist. Such additional perspectives might include things like how the plant makes you feel, what other species associate with it: weather, time of day, phases of the moon and planetary aspects, tutelary deities, dreams, folktales, things that seem similar, and so on. The greater the number and variety of symbol systems that a person can apply to a relationship with a plant—the wider the net, so to speak—the more easily new understandings can be pieced together.

Each new approach, including all the scientific ones, gives us (and the plant) additional vocabulary, more points of contact and connection.

This is why traditional plant people generally welcome new information from science. We are always looking for additional correspondences between the outside world and the human mind, more synonyms for experience. It is not necessary for all the potential meanings available to cohere into a system, only the ones being used. Holding contradictory options open is a good thing, indicating that the bases are covered and that all possibilities have a voice. The more divergent and varied the potential correlations are, the more precise and accurate the conversation and resulting knowledge will be.

For people trained in the scientific method, there are problems with accepting information flowing the other way. Deductive reasoning requires eliminating everything that is subjective, temporary, localized, and contradictory. The useable connections are narrowed to as few as possible (for Galileo, for example, the only important qualities of formerly sacred celestial bodies were weight, density, volume, and present state of motion). The type of information sought is objective—that is, not dependent on the perceiver. It is worth writing down, because it will be just as true tomorrow. It tends to envision systems built out of interchangeable, inanimate parts.

Modern cultures have been guided by the scientific worldview into a set of reductionist, limiting practices that silence nature and make the world appear more solid, immobile, and apparently lifeless than it really is. For example, the many nuances of value expressed in a barter economy far outnumber those possible using money. The synchronization and standardization that results from using one-size-fits-all numerical value systems, like money, clock time, and statistical normalcy, make possible the organization of large groups, such as governments, armies, and corporations. However, the cost of commerce, as fairy tales and poets have consistently warned us, is the loss of the individual's experience of magic—of nature alive and speaking with us.

Although these two worldviews are often contrasted, they are not inherently contradictory. We are people of the modern world, and we must understand standardized systems for our own survival, but it is not necessary to accept them as all that there is, the only valid reality. Here, in our relationships with common plants, we can retain a little undomesticated wildness, a doorway to the dreamtime, a secret garden of the mind where magic can come out and play. Reality expands with our perception of it. Allow the plants to lead you down the garden path, as it were, to fairyland—that fluid and interactive alternate reality that lives within, beside, and beyond objective facts.

THE DOWNSIDE

Being able to speak with nature directly has many benefits, particularly for healers and creative people. However, it is not all pretty flowers and happy songbirds out there. Those who converse with the world as it is must be prepared to acknowledge and process a lot of grief. Plants, being unable to walk away, are far less prone to denial and avoidance than we are. The invasiveness of our own species can't be ignored. The resulting weather disruption, mass extinctions, and other dramatic ecosystem changes are reflected in the experience of the plants. It can be depressing and difficult to see and accept our destructive place in the natural world, and grief is one appropriate emotion; you may experience others. I advise you to move slowly. Sit with what is. Honestly admit your feelings, but be gentle—don't judge; rather, observe. And when you have taken yourself as far as you can, ask the plants for help. They can carry us further. They and their ancestors, the fungi and bacteria, have a lot more experience with evolution than we animals do, and they can teach us things about adaptation when we are ready to learn. They require that, in spite of grief, we appreciate the beauty of the moment as it is, and they offer useful advice, like "bloom anyway." If you have weeds for friends, courage, persistence, and adaptability will develop in you by association.

WIDENING PERCEPTIONS

This expansion of reality is not just a psychological or philosophical concept. It plays out on a physical level as we begin consuming wild plants for food and medicine. Our bodies receive a broad, diverse spectrum of nutrients, minerals, and trace elements, from which our cells access what they need according to the requirements of the moment. They respond with increased abilities to heal, adapt, and realize unexpressed potential.

It is not necessary to live in the wilderness and forage all one's food to benefit from an expansion of the body's capabilities. People who make it a practice to eat three wild leaves a day have noticed increased resilience and stamina. A cup of tea made from herbs freshly picked according to the needs of the time, seeds sprinkled over food, flower garnishes, and foraged condiments add dramatic bursts of color, texture, and flavor to otherwise domesticated meals. These tastes may seem like not much, in terms of volume, but they are packed with wild vitality. Many of the plant compounds that help us heal, shield us from cancer and other disruptions, and enhance general health are diminished or destroyed by heat, overprocessing, and/or storage. Regular consumption of even small amounts of properly prepared fresh wild foods can help counteract many of the ills of civilization and is a great relief to the body. At first, some flavors may seem strong or bitter because they are so concentrated and powerful. You only need a small taste of these, best contrasted with something rather bland. As you become familiar with eating weeds, you may find yourself craving these flavors. Sometimes we may even glimpse the way our animal ancestors grazed according to the opportunities and needs of the moment, allowing scent and taste to guide them in meeting subtly sensed nutritional needs.

FOUNDATIONAL PRINCIPLES

Just as with learning to identify plants, learning to use them is a lifelong process. Some plants are only edible in certain seasons, or only parts of them are edible, or they are only good for food when prepared a certain way. Don't try to do everything at once. Pick a few favorite recipes and techniques and make them specialties of your house. Explore any ancestral traditions you may be aware of, using what is around you. Allow the foods to become bridges. Food may connect past, present, and future, ourselves and our ancestors, and people, homelands, and cultures around the world … everybody eats. However, for these connections and exchanges to be wholesome and effective, rather than exploitive, a few foundational concepts are essential. These principles turn out to be very important in nature. They are not optional. Without them, one can only go so far in getting to know plants, and they will share no secrets.

The first principle is gratitude. Some form of "saying grace" upon harvest, while cooking, and when serving food is believed to increase the body's ability to uptake nutrients. If you haven't inherited a tradition of thankfulness that feels right to you, cultivate your own. It doesn't need to be ornate, and you don't need to believe in anything in particular. All food, but especially foraged food, is a gift from nature, and the knowledge of how to use it is a gift from our ancestors. Say thank you. It's that simple.

Second, eating while those around you go hungry adds a bad taste to any dish. Make it a part of your foraging practice to share goodies. Remember that even small tastes have value. Weeds go very well in stone soup and at potlucks. Take note of those in your community who may not be able to forage for themselves. Find opportunities to share your bounty with children and elders. This is one of the evolutionary lessons that plants teach. Communities that care for all their members adapt to change and resist disaster far better than those that operate on some narrow view of "survival of the fittest." Besides, plants are well known for defining "fitness" differently than society does.

Finally, radical honesty is required, because nature is the ultimate reality check. In the natural world, it is not the thought or intention that counts. Hopes, fears, and fantasies lead to inappropriate actions. The imagination is active when a traditional person is talking with plants, but it is not being used for projections or wishful thinking. It is exploring among the infinite possibilities of truth. The ability to realistically assess our situation and act accordingly is an essential survival technique, one we continually struggle to achieve, both as individuals and as a species. The more we are able to focus our attention on what is actually going on in the present, without judgments and assumptions, the more we open ourselves to participation and understanding... and to joining the conversation.

We tend to think of principles like gratitude, generosity, and honesty in moral terms, as matters of the head and heart, but they find expression on the physical or gut level also. When working with nature, it is best to focus on the physical, biological, tangible aspects of these principles first, as expressed in our actual bodily beings and in our behavior. The rest will follow. Well-nourished, healthy cells lead to a flexible and resilient organism, capable of supporting philosophical prowess (right thinking, sense of beauty) and psychological satisfaction (sanity, happiness). Importantly, also, our physical actions and choices are the substance of our legacy. Whether or not we have children, our existence affects the future. Physically healthy and vigorous plants produce abundant and delicious leaves that feed many other beings; form large numbers of ripe, rich, vital, and viable seeds; and add the most to the compost heap. Whether our "seeds" are offspring, ideas, artworks, or simply the fertility we add to the soil, plants can show us ways to become more delightful and useful citizens of the ecosystem.

NATURAL CYCLES

Let's explore an example of the application of these principles. Beginners often try to focus only on the positive, reject what they dislike, and spread sweetness and light continuously in all directions. However, when contemplating nature with radical honesty, grounded by frequent reference to the physical level of reality, it becomes clear that the world doesn't work that way. The world, in fact, rotates, orbits, and precesses—in other words, it moves in circles.

When we breathe, inbreath and exhale form a continuous cycle, without contradiction or conflict, although they are opposites. When we eat, we excrete, and we are born to die. Breaking, or even interrupting these cycles, inherently leads to imbalance and discomfort. Imagine trying to breathe in but not out. What would that mean for the plants that produce oxygen and depend on exhaled carbon dioxide? Trying to eliminate what seems stale to us removes their refreshment. Any disruption of natural cycles quickly ripples through the webs of life, and the imbalance spreads. This is a disease for which radical honesty is part of the cure. When people are courageous enough to participate fully in all aspects of our personal cycles, facing the truth without judgment, they heal the world from the inside out.

Once honest observation has revealed that our interactions within the material world are all circular, the importance of the other two principles becomes more obvious. Gratitude allows us to fully receive the gifts of life: the inbreath, the feast, the birth of something new, the act of creation. Generosity helps us understand returns: breathing out, releasing, letting go, death and dissolution. Only when all "sides" of a circle are clear of obstacles can it spin smoothly through its phases and seasons for a wholehearted experience.

Radical honesty requires notice of the fact that we move through any and all possible positions around the circumference of those cycles in which we participate. It's quite rare to find ourselves at any kind of axis point or still center. As my mother used to say to us kids, "The world does not revolve around you." This is hard to understand at first, because, of course, our personally perceived world *does* revolve around us. Communing with nature—talking with plants, for example—is one way to open the ability to perceive beyond our immediate sensed human experience and begin to recognize our place in the webs and circles of life.

As living beings, it is natural and right to cling to life. It is proper to struggle against death and dissolution up until the last. Yet this does not mean it is possible to skip, pass over, speed by, or ignore those sections of the circle. When we try, perversions follow, and instead of being a good night, a well-deserved rest, and an honorable and useful ending, death becomes a dreadful void. A glance at the plants quickly gets us out of this muddle. The world does not revolve around us. Our exhales, excrement, and corpses may seem gross, stinky, and disgusting to us, because we are done with them. But they are all a delightful and nourishing bounty to the soil and to the plants, and seeing things from their perspective can change attitudes, and perhaps behavior. It allows us to see some goodness in the night. It encourages gratitude to arise for the life that was not ours by right, but rather a wonderful gift. Generosity may come into play as we consider that which we return as a beneficial offering to the world that has nourished us.

Seeing the cycles of life and death, creation and dissolution from both our own perspective and from that of the plants (and the rest of nature) can be quite steadying. It lets us know that despite our righteous imperative to avoid it, death is not evil. When all sections of the circle are allowed to function, the wheel of time moves smoothly and evenly, and we are more able to deal honestly, generously, and gratefully with all aspects of existence, especially including those parts we would escape if we could, such as the deaths we experience and the deaths we cause.

When we pick a leaf off a plant to eat, we kill that leaf. If we dig a first-year root such as a carrot, we have not only killed that individual, but by harvesting it before it has gone to seed, we have prevented it from fulfilling its life's purpose. Plants, as foundations of the food chain, are notoriously generous in this way. Consider this Buddhist teaching quoted by the Dalai Lama: "May I always be an object of enjoyment / For all sentient beings according to their wish / And without interference, as are the earth / Water, fire, wind, herbs, and wild forests."[2]

Plants understand that the soil in which they grow—in a complex process involving the lives and deaths of many organisms both visible and invisible—is built largely of what was once alive, and that life and death, although opposites, are not in conflict. By cultivating gratitude, generosity, and honesty in our relationships with plants, and by following their lead, we can learn a certain graceful acceptance of the inevitable give-and-take of the cycles of life. Ironically, acceptance of the place of death in the world typically makes people better at survival, more effective and practical, with greater exuberance and zest for life.

Cautions, Warnings, and Risks

"Better safe than sorry."

This expression is often used to support the use of allopathic (modern medical) methods and products—for example, preventive dosing with antibiotics or other drugs. It is also deployed in recommendations against the use of traditional healing plants and other folk medicine. Numerous doctors have told me that since they don't know anything about herbs and their possible interactions, I

---

2. Dalai Lama, *Awakening the Mind, Lightening the Heart* (Dharamshala, India: LTWA, 2008).

shouldn't take them, but should instead rely on the prescription they will write for me. "Better safe than sorry!" they say.

In assessing risk, there is never a clear-cut line between good and bad, safe and sorry. Types of risk have to be balanced. Health involves complex and ever-changing physical, emotional, mental, and spiritual relationships with the rest of the universe, and greater precision and certainty in one area requires more ambiguity somewhere else. Thus, there is not, nor can there be, one right answer to any question, or one right treatment for every person. Each individual, situation, and moment in time calls for a slightly different response. These decisions are very personal. Doctors have to consider liability. We may wish to take other aspects of the larger picture into account, considering the results of our healthcare choices and dietary decisions on issues like animal welfare; economic, environmental, and social impacts; and benefit or harm to future generations. As much as possible, do your own research, including internal research via meditation, prayer, or what is sometimes called soul-searching.

In the example given, the doctors felt sure that their prescriptions were the safest course and assumed that I would agree. Herbs seemed to them to be messy, uncertain, unnecessary, and possibly dangerous. For me, however, herbs are comforting old friends from childhood who have succeeded in helping me many times in the past. Their safe and effective use has been demonstrated and depended upon not only in my family growing up, but in many parts of the world for millennia. They are available for free, grow nearby, and are generally not toxic to the environment when disposed of or excreted. For me, that new pharmaceutical that "just came out" and is heavily advertised to doctors by extremely profitable megacorporations is much more threatening.

Does this mean "never take drugs?" Of course not. I doubt I would be alive today without antibiotics, eyeglasses, and other medical interventions. Does this mean "all the old ways were good?" No. We children, home with the flu, were allowed to play with the mercury from a broken thermometer for hours, until it entirely disappeared. We also enjoyed casting small objects out of lead, which we had melted. We know today that these are not healthful practices, mostly because of what modern medicine has been able to learn through blood tests and other highly technical diagnostic procedures. Frequently the modern and traditional worldviews can be integrated to work together, but sometimes they come into direct conflict. When they do, we have the chance to explore our personal balance of risks and benefits, and find our own dynamic definition of safety.

Let's get specific. There are two plants discussed here: sassafras and comfrey, each of which has a long history of traditional medicinal and culinary use (and in the case of comfrey, agricultural use as a livestock feed). Both plants have been banned as being possibly toxic to the liver. Because of this, it is illegal to sell them, and they are generally no longer recommended for internal use. Reactions from herbalists have run the gamut from "I wouldn't touch them with a ten-foot pole" to "the government is conspiring to steal our power" and everything in between. I have read some of the studies these bans were based on, and I found them underwhelming and unconvincing, especially when stacked up against centuries of indigenous wisdom. I depend upon these two plants, and so I did enough study to feel personally comfortable continuing to rely on them as I always have. It is worth noting that the way I use them does not involve megadoses for a lifetime, nor extracting and refining a single constituent and then injecting it. None of the studies used unstandardized, whole plant compounds seasonally, in moderation, and to taste, as traditional practice recommends. Please do your own research. If you are concerned about a compromised liver, don't drink large amounts of root tea or eat the roots for food. Occasional use of leaf teas should be fine, in my opinion, but I make no recommendations; I ask you to make your own best judgment.

An additional warning concerns allergies. Every so often, someone will be allergic to a common food. Therefore, it is always wise to take only a little the first time you eat any new food, wild or domestic, to see how it sits with you. Be particularly cautious about eating composite flowers (like daisies) if you have pollen allergies. If in doubt, use the petals and not the centers.

Allocation of risk is an area in which we should be making our own decisions, since we will be the ones experiencing the results. If my doctor and I have come to different conclusions about what action to take after saying, "Better safe than sorry," it does not mean that either of us is wrong. It does imply that we both have much to learn, and it gives us a glimpse of exactly how different perspectives on the nature of life lead to wide variations in human behavior, with far-reaching personal and environmental consequences. As stressed at the start, don't eat what you don't know. But also, don't blindly listen to those who fear wildness in general, and foraging in particular. Such a position ignores the entire survival history of our species.

What to Expect

You might say that the first part tells you *why* to forage, and gives a glimpse of the kind of wisdom the plants have to offer, while the classes tell you *how*, complete with harvest times, individual plant portraits, instructions, and tested recipes. Finally, there's an example of intuitive recipe formulation and a discussion of working with a plant's magical and invisible attributes.

Because most of the students from Camp Jabberwocky were beginners, we focused on only a few very widely distributed and easily recognizable plants ... what most people would call weeds. Because we had the plants in front of us, we learned to identify them from life, complete with habit of growth, form, color, taste, and smell. Since I cannot show you the plants, you will need to supplement this book with a good field guide or an experienced teacher if you are making new friends among the weeds.

This book is not designed to teach you to identify the common edibles discussed; instead, the focus is on how to appreciate them, how to approach learning from and about plants, and how to deepen the connections that already exist. It is intended to give you the motivation and tools to put these plants to use once you have found them. I hope that, like me, once you start sampling these wild foods, the many wonderful flavors will draw you in, and the understandings gained from the experience, both rational and intuitive, will enhance your relationships with apparently ordinary plants in delightfully extravagant and magical ways.

Eight Classes

The following chapters are based on eight foraging sessions with Camp Jabberwocky. The focus of each class was on one common and abundant plant. We discussed a theme, brought in other plants relevant to the subject, and asked all kinds of questions, some that can be answered, and some that invite further wondering. Observations of the natural world—what can be noticed—guided these philosophical explorations, becoming party to our exchanges and making them specific and memorable. We were often munching on the featured plant while these conversations were taking place, and eventually we returned to the farm stand to share snacks made of the plant, to swap recipes, and to hydrate, so that the flavors of the plants were an influence, too. The recipes are included here, along with suggestions for a tea or other drink, and each class ends with a practical exercise to deepen perceptive abilities and bring the experience home, or to camp, or wherever we find ourselves next.

Terminology: Common and Latin names

This information will be helpful to you as we move forward. Common or folk terminology is used in this book, because that's the way I was taught. That's fine for working on your own, or with people in your community. When speaking with plants, the important thing is to be honest, clear, and direct, so it is best to use your natural forms of speech and your native tongue. However, if you want to discuss details with other people in other places, it is worthwhile to learn some of the specific technical language that exists in every field.

Latin names are vital for sharing information across cultures. The number of plants called pigweed around the world exceeds a dozen. Plants called myrtle come from thirteen completely different plant families, and I know of four different plants that are called sorrel: the cultivated French kind used in soup; its rangy wild cousin, sheep sorrel, with spearhead-shaped leaves; the wood sorrel, oxalis, a clover look-alike; and the dark red hibiscus flower used for tea in the Caribbean. To avoid confusion when trading recipes and other lore, as well as medicines and seeds, the use of Latin names, which are unique to each plant, will save the day. The first part of the Latin name is the plant's genus, or family group, and the second part indicates the individual species. So, for example, *Amaranthus retroflexus* is the name of the plant I call redroot pigweed, so anyone can distinguish it from all the other plants called pigweed. *Amaranthus* spp. means there are more than one species of the *Amaranthus* family being referenced; for example, when I say that none of pigweed's large family (*Amaranthus* spp.) worldwide is toxic. In the appendix, you will find a list of the common names I have used for the plants mentioned, along with their Latin names and where they come from originally.

A Note on the Recipes

Some of these recipes may seem rambling, almost like stories. That is a sign that they are from a tradition in which recipes (also called

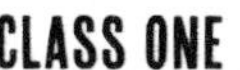

CLASS ONE

Leaves as Foundational Food

Foraging can be intimidating, and I try not to scare off beginners by sending them into the stinging nettle patch right away. It's best to start with something accessible and recognizable that can be seen almost anywhere, anytime—something with a taste most people love: one of the friendly ones. So, at the beginning of the first class with Camp Jabberwocky, we picked and passed around big branches of lamb's quarters for study. Some people are understandably hesitant about eating something new on the word of an odd-looking stranger. Others want to wash it, or photograph it, or get their friend to try it first. Not these campers. As soon as I had eaten a leaf, they began to nibble and graze with enthusiasm. One man said, "I like this," and ate an entire branch. By then

I knew for sure that we would be having some fun together. By the time we returned to the farm stand to try green dip, chilled leftover greens, and pink tea, we had already sampled quite a bit. Once we began grazing as a group, it felt quite natural.

Basic Greens

For most of our development as a species, we have grazed. Primates and other arboreal mammals, while enjoying a wide range of foods, spend most of the time munching on leaves. For predators, another prehistoric (and prehuman) source of greens was fermented, partially digested greens and seeds from the innards of game animals. Animals that eat only meat, like wolves, depend on this source for certain vitamins that meat cannot provide. Recipes based on this ingredient are a delicacy to many people, while the rest of us rely on other fermented foods (see class 7). Whatever the source, green plant material is our foundational food.

Nowadays, our equivalent to grazing is called salad. Basically, anything edible that tastes good "as is" may be tossed into the salad bowl. One benefit of foraging is gaining the ability to enhance salads with a widening variety of additions, increasing with your knowledge, bringing vitality and nutrition as well as diverse flavors, colors, and textures to the mix. Medieval salads included more than a hundred herbs, flowers, and vegetable leaves as well as greens like lettuce and mustard still in use today.

While raw and fermented greens were undoubtedly basic to our original human cuisine, as soon as we had fire and a container of some kind, another iconic dish appeared—the "mess of greens." The recipe is simple. Pick edible greens, wash them, place them in a pot with a little water, and cook them down. A huge volume of leaves is reduced to a dollop of dark green, softened, dense, mild-tasting, more nutritionally complete and available food. The heat and liquid have partially broken down the plant material so that our jaws and digestive systems work less—cooking our greens may possibly even have contributed to the expansion of the brains of evolving humans, as less chewing leads to more talking. All that was very long ago, but greens continue to be a foundational food.

Leaves may be tough or tender, mild, bitter, spicy, or sour. They vary according to season, growing conditions, and age of the plant, generally getting stronger-flavored and more fibrous with time. Quite a few leaves that are tasty as new growth become chewy and bitter as they mature, and the taste of the leaves may change drastically when the plant moves into seed production and begins to flower. Lettuce, for example, goes from mild to very bitter when it sends up its seedstalk and bolts. Dry conditions tend to concentrate flavors. Unless you are in a survival situation, you want to go beyond edibility and arrive at deliciousness. The best way to do this is to keep tasting small bits as you pick. This also has the benefit of letting the plants know that you are grazing. Add a few heartfelt *mmms* and *yums* of appreciation, and the plants will react positively … try it and see.

Keep your method of preparation in mind; some options will concentrate flavors, and others will dilute them. Although drying shrinks plant material and increases intensity that way, volatile flavor oils will evaporate so that leaves lose flavor when dried. Cooking down greens tends to mellow flavors while shrinking volume and creating stock. Boiling greens and then switching out the water for new boiling water one or more times is a way to eliminate bitterness. Nutrients are also poured away with this method, so don't overdo it. However, in the case of some mildly toxic greens, like young poke or milkweed shoots, or greens high in oxalates, which can irritate some people, changing the water can allow indigestible compounds to be poured away, leaving a delightful, tasty, and healthful dish.

Let's talk about bitterness. Certainly, as just mentioned, bitterness can be an indicator of toxicity, a message to the tongue saying, "Don't eat too much of this." We tend to avoid bitterness, gravitating more to sweet and salty flavors. But bitterness has its uses. Having evolved as leaf eaters, our digestive systems have adapted to bypass many of the plant world's defenses. Strong flavors and active compounds in plants like the alliums (onions, garlic, etc.), citrus fruits, and bitter herbs not only fail to repel us, but we have learned to use them to our benefit—that is, medicinally. Bitter herbs stimulate us to be able to digest what would otherwise be difficult or harmful to eat: not only mild toxins and indigestible compounds in plants, but also animal fats and rancid meat and fish. Having spent much of our development as a species as omnivorous scavengers, we can digest a much wider range of foods than the specialists. This versatility requires that we have relatively long digestive systems filled with incredibly diverse organisms capable of a wide range of actions under changeable conditions. So how do we know what to deploy, and when? The taste of bitterness indicates that it's time to "turn on the digestion—full alert."

In the days before refrigeration and canning—especially in circles where rich food was available and overeating was an option, and also for those whose "sensitive digestions" were not accustomed to rich food—small doses of bitter herbs extracted in alcohol provided "aperitifs" before a feast that made everything more digestible. Many cuisines traditionally serve rich meat with bitter or spicy condiments that provide a digestive stimulant, such as pickles, mustard, or horseradish. Bitter drinks like coffee are served after the meal as well, all in the interests of good digestion.

The ability to taste bitterness is quite variable from person to person, depending on genetics and the requirements of the digestive system. It also changes for the individual over time—our sense of taste alters significantly at puberty and again in elderhood. It's important to realize that young children are very sensitive to bitter flavors, strong medicines, and toxins, and can tolerate far less of them than the adults around them. The stereotype of the child who will not eat spinach is based in developmental biology, and such a child should not be forced … if not turned against them by early unpleasantness, strong-flavored greens may still become a healthy and desirable adult favorite. A good way to avoid greens that are too strong for your current taste is to sample as you pick. You may also include small amounts in food that is otherwise overly bland.

The number of different plants that are used for salads and potherbs is staggering. I will mention three families of plants that are foraging favorites—some of the most prolific and delicious in our area: lamb's quarters, the amaranth family, and mustard greens. They are all non-natives that have made themselves at home here, and so they are most common in disturbed areas such as gardens, roadsides, and farmland. These are in a class of foraged foods called pot-stuffers or hunger-chasers; they tend to be nourishing and abundant enough to be staple foods. Tasty and versatile, in general they are used raw when small and tender, and cooked thereafter. All are valued for both leaves and seeds in their places of origin, and together, they can "stuff a pot" and feed a crowd.

Plant Portrait: Lamb's Quarters
(Chenopodium album)

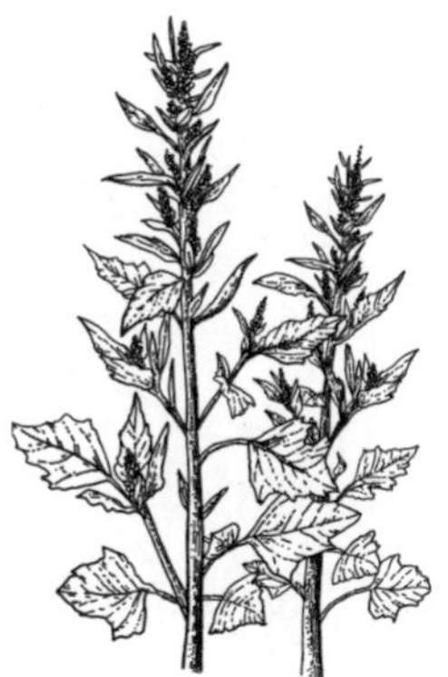

Like the Jabberwocky campers, someone new to foraging might also wish to begin with lamb's quarters. It is a very adaptable plant, so it may be found growing under a wide range of conditions, although not usually as tall and lush as it grows in the garden. Of the three families discussed here, lamb's quarters is the mildest in flavor, and it has the least tendency to become bitter with age. It is also the easiest to identify, with its distinctive gray-green color and mealy texture, making the leaves look somewhat frosted, especially on their undersides and on new growth. It tastes rich, somewhat like spinach, because it is unusually densely packed with vitamins and minerals. To me, a dish of tender young lamb's quarters is superior to any cultivated green.

Lamb's quarters is also an accessible food in terms of method. There are no toxic or inedible parts, no secrets or tricks for harvesting and cooking; it is good raw or cooked, and any spinach recipe will give you a starting point in its preparation.

Plant Portrait: The Amaranths

(Amaranthus spp.)

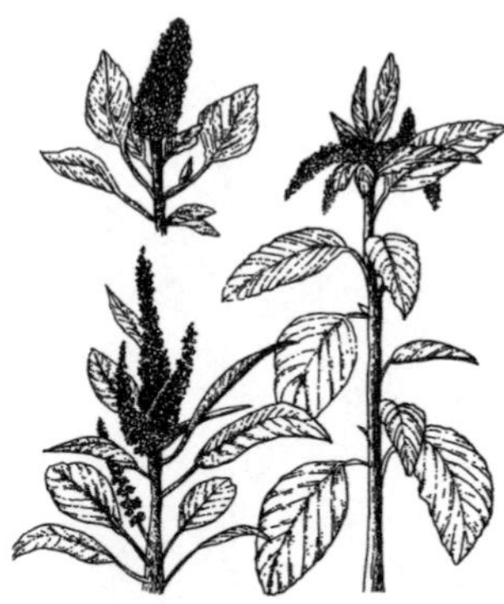

This prolific family produces impressive amounts of palatable and nourishing greens. There are a number of wild forms, and many varieties have been bred for leaf production, for their seeds, or as ornamentals. As a result, there's a lot of variation in their appearance, and to a certain extent in flavor, but all are edible. All may be sampled raw, and are used as salad greens when very young, and as cooking greens thereafter, until they become too tough. Although best in spring, some tender tips can usually be harvested throughout the growing season.

The common wild amaranth here is redroot pigweed. Other varieties have been planted and allowed to seminaturalize; some always go to seed, and when spring comes, the young seedlings get transplanted into a suitable spot. Easiest to identify are the many bright or dark red varieties. They include ornamentals like celosia, elephant's head, and love lies bleeding; some of the types grown for grain; and Hopi red dye, traditionally used to color ceremonial corn bread. Like beet greens or a favorite tea herb, purple basil, amaranths turn any food or brew a gorgeous pinky-red shade. This vivid coloring adds zing to dishes that might look pale and uninteresting, and is noticeably appetizing with berry teas, seeming to accentuate their flavors with visual reinforcement. They add pleasant flavors and nutrition of their own as well.

Plant Portrait: Mustard Greens
(Sinapis and Brassica Families)

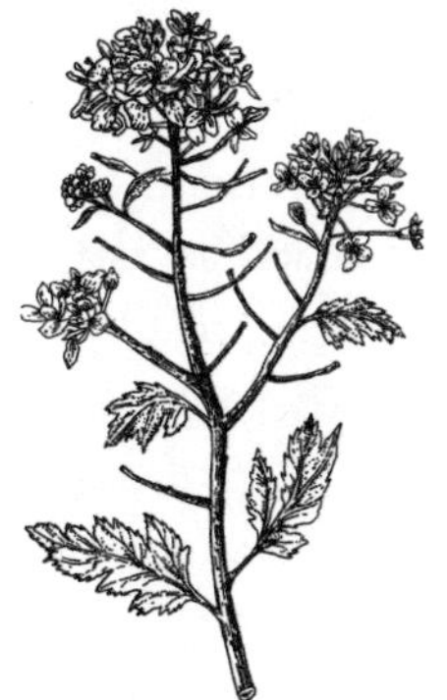

Mustard greens are beloved by many cultures for their flavor and their healthful properties. Like the amaranths, there are many varieties, both wild and cultivated, and they have a tendency to cross and naturalize easily. Start with a few that are common in your area ... here, that would include black mustard and field mustard or charlock. Like the amaranth family, the different mustards can look quite different from one another, but they all have that characteristic spicy flavor when raw. When young and tender, they make a zingy addition to salads, and picking the small leaves and flowering tips is a favorite way to decorate salsas, curries, tacos, and other spicy foods. As they mature, they tend to get hotter and harsher in flavor, and when they have become too strong to enjoy raw, it's time to switch over to cooking them, first in stir-fries and braises, and later boiled down as a potherb in a mess of greens or in soups and stews. They mellow considerably in flavor when they are cooked.

List: Dressing Greens

All around the world, greens both cooked and raw are most often dressed with a combination of grease and something sour, often fermented. This is a great flavor combination, helping to cut any bitterness in the greens, but there is more to it. Part of why it tastes so good is that this combination of fat, acid, and plant material causes the nutrients in the greens to become significantly more bioavailable and accessible to the body ... more digestible. These nutrients include volatile vitamins like the Bs and Cs (especially if raw or only lightly cooked) and minerals like iron and calcium, as well as a constellation of trace elements reflective of the soil in which they were grown, contributing unique flavors of the region—what the French call *terroir*. It is flavor that guided our ancestors in preparing the most nutritious meals as well as the most delicious ones. Is there a recipe in your cuisine that follows this widespread ancient pattern? Think of these classic flavorings when dressing greens:

- bacon grease, hambone, or other smoked meat, with vinegar and hot sauce
- sesame oil, sherry or sake, soy sauce

- mustard oil, tamarind, pickled lime
- mayonnaise and other egg-based sauces
- vinaigrette, oil and vinegar-based salad dressings
- butter, wine, lemon, capers
- sour cream or yogurt

Greens Recipes

These recipes may be made with any kind of foraged greens, as well as cultivated greens like spinach, kale, and collards. Most traditionally, they are made with a mess of greens: a mixture of whatever looked best when you went out to pick. For the leaf crisps, it's best to use leaves of similar thickness, but most recipes benefit from mixing multiple species for both flavor and ease of picking. As you expand your knowledge of edible plants, you will be able to add more and more diversity to your salads and messes of greens.

Recipe: Leaf Crisps

Some people who don't like greens in other forms will munch on these ... and making leaf crisps in the dehydrator is a good class project. I recommend starting with plantain, but any leaf you would eat raw can be used. Here are some tips:

- wash and dry the leaves well
- remove thick stems
- toss with a SMALL amount of oil ... just a few drops
- spread in a layer one leaf thick on a cookie sheet or dehydrator rack
- use low heat; 250 degrees Fahrenheit in the oven or a dehydrator both work well
- once they are crisp, cool for three minutes and serve
- I like them plain, but if you want to add soy sauce, salt, spices, and so on, do it after cooking

Recipe: Green Yogurt

Here is a versatile dip, sandwich spread, or filling for stuffed flowers, leaf rollups, cherry tomatoes, and so on.

- 1 cup of cooked greens, coarsely chopped, drained, and pressed dry
- 1 quart of plain whole milk yogurt
- salt to taste

Line a sieve or colander with a damp cloth and set over a bowl. Allow the yogurt to drain for an hour (for dip) or overnight in the fridge (for a stiffer mixture suitable for spread or filling). Mix in greens and salt to taste. Serve chilled or at room temperature.

Variations:

- any combination of greens may be used (I like lamb's quarters and pigweed)
- sub out some of the drained yogurt for sour cream, cottage cheese, or ricotta
- add garlic, green onion, lemon zest, or other herbs and spices as desired
- garnish with flowers and/or add flower petals to the mix

Recipe: Leftover Greens

I never measure when I make this, estimating according to the quantity of greens I have left over. You can do the same, using this recipe as a guide to proportions.

- 1 cup of cooked, very well-drained greens
- 1 teaspoon of soy sauce or tamari
- 1 teaspoon of vinegar, preferably rice or balsamic
- ½ teaspoon of toasted sesame oil
- 1 splash of hot sauce, or to taste

Toss to blend and refrigerate overnight. Eat the next day, ice-cold. This dish is so good it's worth making leftovers on purpose.

Beverage: Sun Tea

- a small handful of lemon balm
- a few red clover blossoms
- a sprig or two of red amaranth (any kind)

To make sun tea, try a favorite blend of herbs like this one, or pick a handful of leaves or a tea bouquet according to the whim of the moment. Place them in a glass vessel with a lid. I use a gallon jar, but a quart will work also. Fill with warm or cool water, cover, and let steep all morning in the hot sun. By afternoon, the tea should be colorful and flavorful. It's good served warm, cool, or iced.

Practice: Three Wild Leaves

You might be interested in trying the practice of eating three wild leaves a day. It is not the habit of most modern people to just munch leaves from a bush as you pass by, graze off the lawn, or chomp on flowers, but it is very satisfying when you have become used to it. Of course, you will make sure the leaves you choose are clean, fresh, and of an edible variety. Once you have developed a taste for something (as I have for the spicy little yellow floral fireworks of the charlock or field mustard), you begin to notice them here and there, the way city people notice restaurants, markets, or vending machines. Even if you do not choose to eat from them at this time, you know where food is, and that is a comforting feeling.

Leaves, like fruit, are a part of the plant that is designed to be eaten. Leaves are relatively expendable compared to the other plant parts and are more quickly replaced. At some points in a plant's annual cycle, it may even be beneficial for the plant to be pruned by grazing and foraging in order to develop the root system, and not coincidentally, these are the times the leaves are the most tender and taste best, without bitterness.

Many traditional healers and plant people report that the plants a person needs most will grow around them, or grow with particular lushness, or in some way attempt to reach out (sometimes literally) to the one in need. If a certain plant is following you around, appearing before you unexpectedly, or presenting in your dreams, it might be wise to look into what that plant may be trying to say or bring to you. If it is edible, eating three leaves a day is an easy and natural form of communion. If it's not, or if you don't know, do some research, and you may find that what you discover will have some special or necessary meaning for you. Don't assume that all the choosing, learning, intention setting, and conversations are directed by or originating with you. Allow some room for those plants that have something to offer you to reveal and express themselves. Making it a regular habit to eat three wild leaves provides an opportunity for you to be reached out to, just in case.

List: Ways to Use Leaves

- dried or fresh as a seasoning
- tea
- young and fresh in salads and as garnish
- cooked down
- shredded and marinated in vinegar or citrus
- braised, sometimes with stalks and buds
- stir-fried
- steamed
- tempura
- fermented or pickled
- soups and stews
- casseroles

- smoothies
- green salsa, dips, pesto, and spreads
- edible wrappers for steamed, baked, or grilled foods
- baked, grilled, or dehydrated chips
- herb butters, infused oils

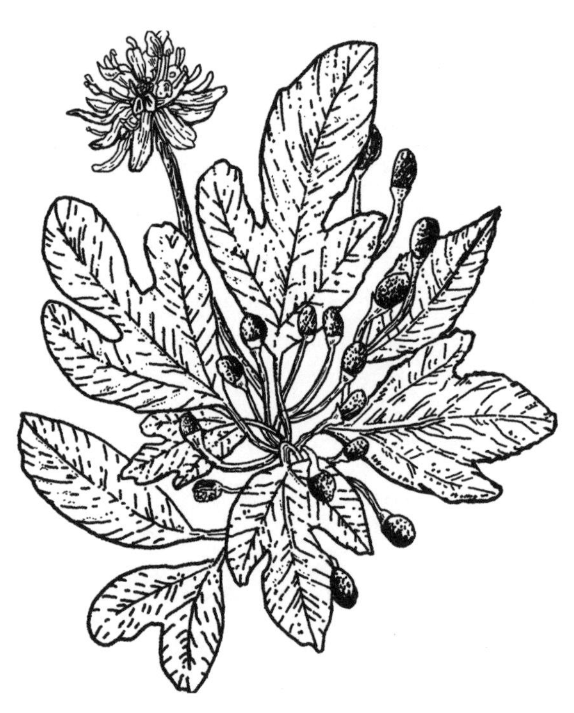

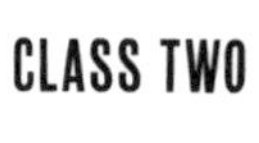

CLASS TWO

Roots, Seeds, and Sprouts

On the day we discussed the history of the farm, we were watching the brilliant and acrobatic goldfinches eating seeds from the swaying weed stalks. We admired the connections between past and future that living beings embody as we each individually channel and express our shared inheritances. We considered some of the ways that traits and relationships change over time, for plants and places as well as for birds and people. The various parts of plants have different qualities and flavors according to the changing seasons, and we examined some typical harvest cycles, while recognizing that each species has its own quirks and tendencies. Here are some tips for wholesome harvests, digesting history, foraging roots, a sprinkling of seed recipes, and some fun and interactive games with sprouts.

History and the Future

Roots and seeds are complimentary opposites, like inbreath and exhale, or dawn and dusk. When plants are taken as metaphors, teachers, or examples for humans, our lives may be seen as briefly rising from the roots of an ancestral past to fling seeds far beyond our reach, into the future. Roots are associated with beginnings and with one's original place; when a seed sprouts, its first vital effort is the emergence of the anchoring taproot.

When speaking of individuals and cultures, our ancestors and their homelands, traditions, and ways are our anchoring roots. The stories of our elders ground and nourish us. It is said that the depth and firmness of our foundational roots determine the extent of our reach outward and upward, toward the sun and stars. We can strengthen and expand this root system through attention and exercise, by sending awareness down, and by eating the roots of plants as we tell the old tales. It is the strength of the root system that allows young sprouts to take new directions, to grow into new space and greater light for the benefit of the entire organism, roots included.

All the same, roots are limiting. They are what connect and confine us to this time, this place, and this life. Here we make our stand,

and make our choices. Here we draw our nourishment and the water of life, and here we leave the gift of our "parts" to be recycled when we die. The uniqueness of each lifetime grows and changes and passes away in the here and now, and each individual finds the conditions different and unrepeatable. Beyond this present situation we cannot go.

History and our relations with our forebearers can be both a help and a hindrance. We don't want to perpetuate the evils and errors of the past, and we strive to rectify them. Yet we want to remain true to our roots, and to honor our ancestors as they deserve—despite shortcomings, they made it possible for us to be here. So how do we sort through our heritage? Shall we carry forward the family recipes and leave behind the offensive jokes? What about those odd, ancient, gruesome fairy tales? Some deeply rooted connections, it seems, are not easy to lose. Ideally, we could appreciate and learn from our ancestors, drawing from their experience and beliefs without being limited by them as we navigate a way forward into uncharted territory.

When a plant goes to seed, it is able to send itself beyond the reach of its roots in both time and space. The prolific annual weeds that provide the bulk of my foraged food, like lamb's quarters, amaranth, chickweed, and purslane, bear very hard shelled seeds in great quantities. These tiny seeds will germinate on and off for more than forty years, and the plants that grow from them will express a wide range of the species' capabilities. Who knows what will be asked of them out there in the distant future? From an evolutionary point of view, it's best not to require descendants to be too much like the parents, but to allow as much diversity as is physically possible. In our seeds are stored the best of what we know from the past, and our best guesses about what will be needed in the seasons to come—plus a few wild cards, just in case. Seeds are hope with a hard shell.

Because seeds contain such concentrated vitality, they make desirable food, especially since they can be stored for long periods of time ... assuming they can be protected from thieves, rodents, insects, and spoilage. The need to securely store grass seed was a major driver in the development of pottery, stone buildings, and standing armies. Grain has been called one of the foundations of civilization. Today, we still rely on civilization and machinery to produce, process, and distribute grass seeds like wheat, corn, and rice, which are staple foods around the world. Many lesser-known seeds and grains surround us. Some of the culinary weeds, like the amaranths and plantains, are valued commercially for their seeds, and many beloved spices are seeds, too. Although they may be time-consuming to harvest and prepare, the density of the life force and nutrition seeds provide is unsurpassed.

A seed has within itself the nourishment necessary to start a plant growing. This usually includes proteins, healthy oils and oil-soluble vitamins, and a range of minerals reflecting those in the soil in which it grew. Most seeds come enclosed in a coating that shelters the tender germ where sprouting begins. This allows them to wait in the soil without rotting until conditions are right for growth. It also allows many of them to pass through the digestive tracts of animals, birds, and insects, to emerge somewhere new, wrapped in fertilizer and full of potential. When we creatures excrete some of those seeds, this naturally causes the tastiest of our staple food plants to grow more abundantly around us—the first form of agriculture. To encourage this method of dispersal, many plants have made eating their seeds delicious and attractive, placing them inside of fruit, for example. However, to benefit from the nutrition within the seed itself, the outer shell must be breached. Toasting, steaming, boiling—exposure to heat can crack the shell. Soaking, fermentation, sprouting—liquids may be used to soften the husk. Chewing, grinding, pounding—making meal or flour uses pressure to break open the seeds. When relatively basic technology is used, enough intact seeds will often slip through to serve the plant's reproductive purposes.

The majority of a plant's life's work eventually dies to become compost and feed the life of the soil, on which future fertility for newly rooting seedlings will depend. Annuals perform this sacrifice yearly, biennials take two years, and perennials do the same over a longer period of time. All the parts that used to be essential for survival—stalk and stem, leaves, flowers, and even roots—are relinquished, and potential is carried forward as seeds alone. Observe the courage and adaptability required by these plants that must first die back almost completely, and then use whatever they find around them to completely regrow new versions of themselves. They emerge ready to undertake the traditional ancestral dance in a new season, under unpredictable conditions of weather and climate, from a position of freshness and delight… and that tenderness and enthusiasm is part of what makes them delicious. As a result of this daring strategy, these plants are weeds: common and always ready to grow, wherever conditions are favorable, now and far into the future.

As we evaluate our own various cultural inheritances, we might take cues from these evolutionary lessons, and ask ourselves what an unknown future might require. In general, the ability to dream—combined with flexibility, creativity, curiosity, and skills and techniques for experimentation—seems more useful than loyalty to a fixed past. The adaptability shown by the plants we forage is also required of us, as each generation works out what to pass along, what to renew, and what to leave behind. It's a continuous process, naturally uneasy, with a lot of ambiguity and uncertainty built in.

As complementary opposites, both roots and seeds are necessary and essential. We respect and care for our roots that have allowed us to survive and continue to support us, while in the long run, it's the formation of seeds—whatever we send beyond our individual lives into the future—that steers our species on its evolutionary course. When in doubt, honor the roots, and favor the seeds. Look for the anchors and the hard-shelled hopes, and for what will be useful. Plants don't mourn the past, or deny, rewrite, or try to hold on to it. Instead, they break it down, digest it, and absorb its complex components … the past is the future's food.

Plant Portrait: Sassafras
(Sassafras albidum)

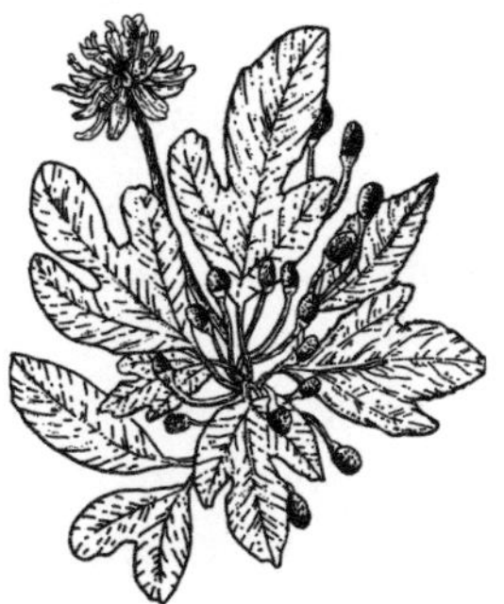

If you want to taste some powerful history, find a grove of sassafras trees. They like moist woodlands and field edges, spread by sending up suckers to form clumps, and bear a blue two-seeded drupe (like a berry) that is carried to new places by birds.

Sassafras is an easily and definitively recognizable plant—no other tree has three differently shaped leaves. There's the oval, the three-lobed, and the mitten-shaped leaves, all on the same tree, sometimes all on the same branch. Its growth habit is distinctive, both the way it grows in colonies and the patterns formed by the way the branches join the trunk. In winter, it is most easily recognized by the bark: brown and deeply ridged on the trunk; brown, freckled, and somewhat coarse on the larger branches; and bright green and freckled on the smaller branches. The smallest twigs may be bright green and entirely smooth. One of these small green twigs may be used as a toothbrush; chew on it awhile and enjoy its breath-freshening flavor. Don't forget to mentally or verbally ask permission, and leave a small gift with your thanks, whether the answer is yes or no. Once you have met the sassafras tree, you will be able to confirm your ID even in the dark by recognizing its strong and distinctive scent and taste.

Sassafras root and bark were New England's second largest export to Europe in the early days of colonization, after tobacco. Like tobacco, sassafras was considered a new "wonder drug" and used as a general tonic and to treat diseases from the "new world," especially syphilis. Sassafras root tea is a traditional spring tonic and is the main flavor in root beer, which was originally a healing beverage made at home and used as medicine, especially in the early spring hunger times when stored food ran low and few fresh foods were available. To make root beer, a strong tea is sweetened and allowed to ferment slightly, just until it gets fizzy, so that while the alcohol content is still low (2–3 percent), the probiotic content is very high. Usually, a combination of health-enhancing flavorful roots was used, including sassafras and ginger, calamus, sarsaparilla, elecampane, and many more.

During the summer, a tea of twigs and leaves, simmered gently awhile, makes a refreshing drink, hot or cold. It may be sweetened, flavored, and colored by adding a few crushed ripe berries as it cools.

A classic culinary ingredient made from sassafras leaves is the bright green powder called filé (pronounced *FEE-lay*), which is the signature ingredient in filé gumbo, creating a flavorful, gummy sauce. The "slimy" texture of this thickener is not for everyone, but okra lovers will probably take to it right away. Filé gumbo is a combination dish, originally made with all foraged ingredients by Cajun (French Acadian) people who were driven from their homeland by violence and had to resettle in a place where the environment was totally different. The recipes and traditions that arise when old cooking techniques combine with new ingredients have historically produced some of the world's most iconic dishes, and filé gumbo is one of them.

To make filé, pick young, fresh-looking leaves, dry them in the shade until crisp, and powder them. For a small amount, rub between the hands and pick out the strands that come from the large veins in the leaves. For larger quantities, rub the dried and crumbled leaves through a sieve or grind them on a stone or mortar, or in a blender. Filé powder is added after cooking is complete, or it may be sprinkled on at the table; do not boil your dish after adding filé, or the texture will not be as nice.

The Cajuns and other resettlers, of course, learned about sassafras and other foods and medicines in their new homes from the native people who had already been living there. (In the case of the Wampanoag on Martha's Vineyard, for about eleven thousand years.) The sort of land knowledge that develops over such a long period of time is very powerful. That is one reason, along with the theft of fertile land, why so many tribes were "relocated" to unwanted areas in unfamiliar territory. People often remark on the special, magical, healing properties of Cape Cod and Martha's Vineyard. Not everyone knows that one reason for that undefinable quality of rightness is the presence of modern native people living on their ancestral homelands. Much has been lost as well as gained over the course of the centuries, but one thing that has not been forgotten is the smell and taste of sassafras.

Cultural shifts may give rise to great recipes, but they are hard on the people living through them. Sassafras has a long-lived reputation as an adaptogen and tonic; that is, a medicine that helps people adjust to the stresses of life and extreme change. As we attempt to shift our own cultures toward more realistic, just, and survivable ones, the sassafras tree with its fortifying flavor and tonic medicine is an old ally with plenty of spirit, stamina, and resilience.

Eating Seeds and Roots

Most roots are not as easy to identify as those of sassafras. It will probably take a while to become familiar with them. It can take several seasons of observation to piece together the different plant stages, with roots and seeds being the hardest to identify. Usually you will recognize the leaves, flowers, and fruits first. This process can be sped along by taking pictures of the same plant through the seasons. Of course, once you have eaten a lot of anything, it becomes familiar, just as experienced cooks can tell carrots, turnips, potatoes, and parsnips apart at the market. Until then, take your time, and make sure of your identification. Toxic roots and bulbs do exist—daffodils, for example, and some wild carrot relatives. Beware also of poison ivy roots, with their little hairy brown rootlets—they can give you a rash just like the rest of the plant.

Once observation has made you confident of the plant's identification, the next issue is timing. The roots we favor for food are the big fat ones, used by the plant to store energy in the form of starches and sugars, as well as to absorb energy in the form of nutrients and water from the soil. It makes sense that the tastiest and most nutritious roots are those harvested when the most energy is stored there. By following the plant's life cycles, we can guess when and where to seek peak nutrition and flavor.

ANNUALS: An annual completes its life cycle in one year, sprouting, growing, flowering, fruiting, and going to seed, then dying. It will not regrow from the old root, but new plants will emerge from the numerous seeds. It will go to seed under the most adverse conditions, because it only has the one chance. The best time to dig the roots of annuals is when they have sized up but before the plants send up their flower stalks and switch over to bloom mode. Radish is a common garden example that often naturalizes here. Most annuals are used more for greens than for roots; because annual plants don't require energy storage over the winter, their roots tend to be scrawny.

BIENNIALS: A biennial plant takes two years to complete its life cycle. The first year it forms a low rosette of leaves but no flowers or seeds. The top dies back over the winter, but has stored its life underground. The next year it sends up one or more stalks of flowers, forms fruits or pods, and goes to seed before dying off completely. These stalks are often quite magnificent, having the benefit of two seasons' preparation. The seeds tend to be large and elaborate and packed with beneficial oil-soluble nutrients. Biennials store a lot of energy in their roots after the first summer, and although some energy gets expended in surviving the winter, most of it is being saved for sending up the flower stalk in the second year, so they're excellent in the fall of the first year and still very good the following spring. Once they begin their second season's growth and become recognizable by the flower, the root has gotten stringy, woody, and tough; it is no longer a storage area, although it's still doing duty as an anchor and conduit. Evening primrose, garlic mustard, and the docks are examples of biennial roots.

PERENNIALS: A perennial is a plant that comes back year after year from the same root system. Some persist for only a few years; others can live for a century or more. Most produce seeds yearly; often the quality and quantity of these seeds depend a lot on that season's weather, with some "bad" years producing little or no seeds, as the plant waits for better conditions by retreating to the roots. The flow of sap in trees is an example of the way the life force moves through perennial plants. Usually, the roots are best in the fall and early spring. Dandelion is a perennial.

If you simply follow the flavor, the plant will tell you when to eat which part of it and where the best nutrition can be found. We let goats into the community garden at the end of the season so they can eat down the weeds before the winter's cover crop is planted. First, they fight over any especially delectable remains, such as bean vines. After that, they set about carefully stripping the grainy seed heads off each and every stalk, and they will not go back and eat the stalks themselves until all the seeds are gone.

Seed Recipes

The large family that provides us with spicy mustard greens also produces spicy seeds, which can be used in many ways. The amaranths produce tasty seeds, as do lamb's quarters, plantain, dock, and many others. As with greens, you can harvest one kind or mix them according to availability and taste. The best way to harvest is usually to pick or cut the whole seed head and hang a bundle of heads upside down in a paper bag. As the seed heads dry, the seeds will drop into the bag. How thoroughly you clean them after that depends on your recipe and your taste; it is not harmful to include some chaff and bits of stem and leaf in crackers or cereal, for example. These are method recipes, meant to use however many seeds you have at hand, from a small handful to a large bucketful.

Recipe: Mustard Sauce

Toast (optional) and grind mustard seeds, any kind or a combination. Add a little water or vinegar to make a paste, as coarse or fine as you like. Store in the fridge.

Recipe: Seed Sprinkle

Toast and partially crush seeds, one type at a time, and then combine them. Use as a condiment, or add to dressings, dips, salads, and salsas for flecks and crunch similar to coarsely ground black pepper, although with different flavors.

Recipe: Seed Crackers

Roll out bread dough fairly thinly onto a sheet of parchment paper. Any dough from a rich brioche (crumbly) to a lump of plain pizza dough (crisp) will be good—sourdough is excellent, and pie crust works, too. Press seeds into the surface if the dough is sticky enough, or brush with butter or beaten egg white to glue on the seeds. You may use one type of seed, or mix them, or put each type of seed on its own section of dough for a single batch of assorted crackers. Place the paper and dough on a baking sheet and cut into strips, diamonds, or squares with a pizza cutter or dull knife, or cut out shapes with a cookie cutter. Bake in a hot oven (400 to 450 degrees Fahrenheit) until just beginning to brown around the edges. Cool and store airtight.

Recipe: To Toast Seeds

For small amounts, a skillet works well. Keep the seeds moving and toss frequently, until they begin to pop and release their aroma: three or four minutes, depending on the size and dryness of the seeds. For larger amounts, spread the seeds shallowly in large baking pans in a 350-degree-Farenheit oven and stir often, keeping a close eye on them for the last few minutes. I recommend toasting each variety of seed separately and then combining them. Toasted seeds make good additions to granola, snack mixes, and cookies.

Recipe: Porridge

This classic ancestral dish is found in various forms around the world. Seeds may be left whole or soaked, toasted or cracked, then they are simmered in liquid until they are tasty and digestible. Porridge is generally used as a bland base for flavorful toppings, and leftovers make a useful addition to baked goods and casseroles.

Recipe: Sprouts and Microgreens

Seeds from lamb's quarters or amaranth or any other plant whose leaves are edible may be sprouted and eaten whole, using any method recommended for alfalfa, mung beans, or other domesticated sprouts. My personal preference is to plant the soaked seeds in a small amount of potting soil and cut small leaves as they grow. Sometimes called microgreens, these small leaves can add a lot of zing to a winter dish.

Recipe: Flourless Seed Brittle

This makes enough to spread on one baking pan. Combine one cup of flaxseeds, three tablespoons of chia seeds, a half cup of ground flax, and a half to three-fourths cup of other seeds, such as sunflower, evening primrose, or any combination of edible seeds you like. Mix with three cups water and a half cup of pickle juice, or use all water and add half a teaspoon of salt or one tablespoon of tamari or soy sauce. Allow seeds to soak for at least two hours or overnight. Spread on parchment paper on a cookie sheet and bake in 250 degrees Fahrenheit for one hour or a little more, then leave to cool in the oven. Alternatively, put the parchment paper in a food dehydrator and let it run until the brittle is hard. It should be very crisp. Broken up and stored airtight at room temperature, this crunchy treat will keep for a month. It's very high in fiber, so be sure to accompany the brittle with plenty of liquids.

Recipe: Historical Seaweed Cakes

This recipe is based on an ancient dish from the Stone Age that is still popular in Wales. Originally cooked on the bakestone, today it is usually made on a wrought iron pan or electric griddle.

Gather wild oats and other edible seeds or use oatmeal (not the quick-cooking kind). Toast on the bakestone, in a pan, or in the oven. Stir often. The oats should dry out and just begin to brown. Cool and grind in a mortar, on a grindstone, or in a blender or food processor. Sift if necessary to remove husks. Any toasted oat flour, from coarse and branny to a fine silky powder, will work well.

In Wales, this recipe is made with laverbread, which is a type of very firm dark purple seaweed with thin fronds; it grows on the rocks where little bivalve shellfish called cockles are also collected. Here we don't have laverbread, so other seaweeds must be used. If the seaweed is tough, like laverbread or kelp, stew it in a slow cooker with a tablespoon or two of lemon juice until it is soft. This can take hours if the seaweed is very solid. Delicate seaweeds like dulse and sea lettuce are also good, and do not need precooking. If fresh, rinse at the last minute, and only if necessary to remove sand. Chop as finely as possible by hand or by machine. If dried, soak several hours or overnight, squeeze out as much liquid as possible (the liquid is a salty and nutritious broth, which makes a useful base for soup). The end result should be a soft, loose, gelatinous mush.

Mix toasted oat flour with the drained seaweed until you reach the consistency of a thick, somewhat sticky paste. Pat into little flat cakes, any size you like—I use walnut-sized pieces, but some make them larger. Cook on a very hot, well-greased griddle, pan, or stone. Bacon grease is preferred in Wales, duck or goose fat is also very good, but any grease you would use to fry an egg will do. Fry like croquettes, browning on both sides. Traditionally a breakfast food, try them also for a salty, savory snack or side dish packed with history, nutrition, and plenty of flavor.

Recipe: Easy Seaweed Cakes

Soak half a cup of dried dulse overnight; drain and press until mostly dry. Toast one cup of noninstant oatmeal until just browned and whiz in a blender to a medium-coarse flour.

Mix and let set for five minutes, then fry in butter or grease. This makes two servings.

Fun with Sprout Crafts

A sprout is a bridge between the seed and the root, containing elements of both. They are plants in the process of moving beyond their past and the genetic expectations of their ancestors, and reaching into the future in which they will live out their particular individual lives, and to which they will commit their own seeds if they can. This makes them ideal allies for transitional work.

Seeds that sprout easily can be used to make interesting creations that change over time. Art projects using sprouts are limited only by your ingenuity. Grasses like rye and various kinds of lawn grass or hayseeds work well, as do plantain, amaranth, or mustard seeds. If you want to try one of these projects and have not collected your own seeds, you may use store-bought psyllium, flax, or chia if they are fresh and whole.

Seeds on something damp and absorbent will sprout and grow for a while using only water and the energy that is in the seed. Grow them on anything that is nontoxic and will hold moisture, like unfired clay, cotton balls, scraps of old T-shirts, paper (including paper mâché), cardboard, wool, sponges, a folded cloth, and so on. Of course, a base that holds dirt allows the sprouts to grow bigger, but even so, sprout art does not last. Most sprout artists allow their project to reach an interesting stage and then take pictures. The pictures are the part that can be kept and shared.

Recipe: Pet Treats

Seeds and sprouts from edible plants, like those mentioned above, can be eaten by humans and also dogs, cats, rodents, reptiles, and birds. Caged or indoor pets especially will often appreciate some fresh greens. Just make sure whatever you sprout them on is also edible and won't make a mess. Try sprouting on an organic corncob, or in an extra pet dish.

Craft: Green-Haired Pet

You can make a funny pet better than the ones for sale. Make your pet from anything that can stand to be kept damp for a week or two. An odd sock makes a good base. Stuff with a rag and make a face. Coat with seeds and water to grow fur.

Craft: Mini Plants

Tiny planters and pots (and thimbles and seashells) can be seeded to produce luxuriant houseplants for a dollhouse, model, or miniature scene. In the art of bonsai, *kusamono* (literally "grass thing") is a small seasonal arrangement of grass and flowers.

Craft: Centerpieces or Favors

Grow sprouts in canning jars (or other interesting waterproof containers) until they are slightly more than halfway up the sides. Nestle in a seasonal favor (such as an Easter egg, holiday ornament, or wrapped treat). For place settings, label with the recipient's name. Rye seed makes a good grassy green.

Craft: Absurd Sprout Art

Things you were going to throw away (a broken toy truck, a hairbrush, a raggedy doll, one sneaker, a book, etc.) could look bizarre and interesting with sprouts growing out of them.

Craft: Sprouts Growing in Patterns

A paper plate, piece of cardboard, or other biodegradable base can be covered with a design, or your initials, or some other pattern using glue or paste. Make sure the glue is nice and thick, as seeds are slippery and you don't want them to sprout right away. Dust your design with seeds, shake off lightly, and let dry. When you are ready to sprout, place on an absorbent surface (like a folded paper towel or sponge on a plate) and keep constantly moist. Or, place on a flower pot or tray of soil for a longer-lasting pattern. Another way to make seed papers is to glue the seeds between the folds of a paper napkin. Yet another way is to coat paper dolls, hearts, snowflakes, or other paper shapes with glue and dip them in seeds. You may make seed papers with flower seeds, and they can be planted to grow a bunch of flowers. These make good enclosures in letters or cards.

Craft: Fashionable Sprouts

Hats with patterns of sprouts growing out of them are very nice for fancy garden parties, summer parades, and demonstrations in favor of the environment. Start with a hat you will not want to wear again. Paint with glue, dust with seeds, and keep damp.

Beverage: Root and Bark Teas

Teas made with roots or bark need more heat and time than those made with leaves or flowers. Overheating leaves and flowers drives off the delicate volatile oils that contribute the greater part of their flavors and aromas. Roots, bark, seeds, and other dense and woody materials benefit from being simmered awhile and then allowed to steep a long time, several hours or overnight. Sometimes flavor and nutritional availability are enhanced by roasting the roots before brewing them. Many roots are rich in minerals, such as dandelion, burdock, and sassafras. A piece of root simmering and steeping next to the fire or on the back of the woodstove provides tonic tea for days. Scoop some out to drink, add more water, and continue to steep and simmer until the root stops releasing flavor and color—time to add a new piece of root. Dilute this strong potion until the flavor pleases you. When made in clay or iron pots, additional minerals join the nourishing and tonifying attributes of the roots. Root teas, broths, and soup stocks are generally very nourishing and are particularly known for helping with mineral deficiency symptoms, such as hair loss, skin problems, slow digestion, and lack of vigor.

Practice: Seed Landscapes

(from Dr. Rocio Alarcon G., Curandera)

I learned this practice from a wonderful teacher, Rocio Alarcon G., who is both a curandera from Ecuador and an ethnopharmacologist at the University of London. Like the hummingbird, she flits between worlds, pollinating wherever she lands. This technique has been in her family for generations—it is intellectual property and a valuable inheritance that Rocio has enhanced further. We have permission to share it, but please give Rocio and her grannies credit, acknowledgment, and appreciation whenever this powerful practice is used or shared.

I have a couple of handfuls of mixed seeds rolled up in an indigo-dyed hanky. Every so often, when I have some serious thinking to do, I will spread the seeds out on the cloth or on a wooden tray and stir them around. Sometimes just stirring them is satisfying; at other times, I will arrange and rearrange them into patterns, or sort them by color or size, or mound them into small piles. The knowledge of the future that seeds contain seems to inform my thoughts at such times. Often the answers to questions will arise not long after I have been talking with the seeds. This is also an intriguing practice for children—even very young children can stir beans around in a bowl, and later they may enjoy sorting and counting. If you have the time and space, you may wish to leave the seeds out for a few days, stirring them when you feel like it, or arranging them together with whomever is at the table. There are no rules and requirements; it is the direct contact with the seeds that is important. They don't have to be rare or fancy; my seed bundle contains beans I grew and lentils from the supermarket, because that's what was available, and they work just fine.

List: Ways to Use Seeds

- sprinkled on food
- ground into flour
- as porridge
- in soups, stews, and mixed braises
- whole grains are seeds—add foraged seeds when cooking rice, millet, etc.
- in breads, crackers, energy bars, and cookies
- soaked overnight for pudding or to add to smoothies
- ground into seasoning pastes and sauces
- crispy coatings for fried or baked foods
- sprouts, raw or malted
- ferments and pickles
- pressed for oil
- as spices

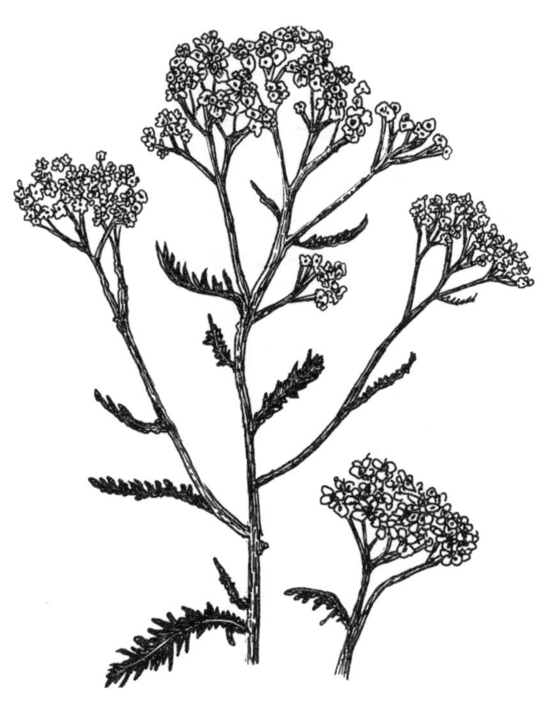

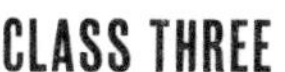

CLASS THREE

Enjoying Invasive Plants

One day, we were playing with month-old goat kids in the shade of the big silver maple. It was a hot and bright day, and the shade, combined with the youthful enthusiasm of the kids, was refreshing. No one wanted to move—goats were climbing into people's laps and playing hide-and-seek among us, particularly enjoying peeking out from under the wheelchairs. Still, the purpose of our gathering was to discuss plants. I looked down, and there at the corner of a community garden was a nice patch of mint, maybe twice the size of a bushel basket. How delightful! We had our plant visit on the spot.

Plant Portrait: Mint
(Mentha spp.)

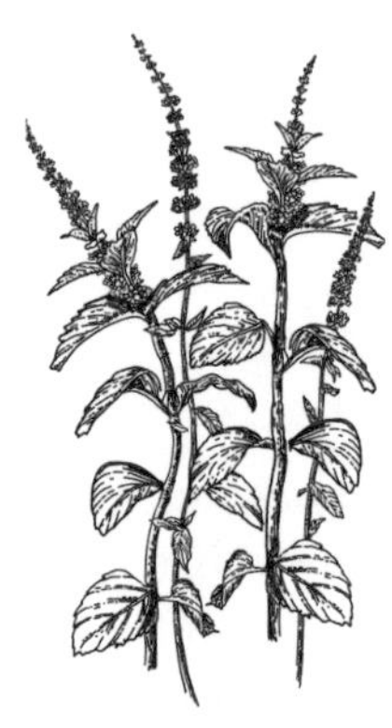

This patch of mint was growing half inside the garden, where it had been planted in a pot but had escaped, and half outside the fence, where we could easily pick and taste it. Both halves were equally tall and vigorous, indicating that goats, deer, and poultry would not eat it. Well into a hot, dry summer it looked lush and pristine, showing that bugs didn't fancy it either, and that the tangled mats of spreading rhizomes were very water efficient. The spreading nature, and the fact that nothing was growing in with it, tipped us off that we were looking at an invasive plant. We recalled the enormous patch of horehound, another member of the family, that has taken over a corner of the far field, a legacy of another community gardener. To confirm, the goats turned up their furry noses at the mint we offered.

We, however, enjoyed the fragrance and flavor, and we rubbed and sniffed and nibbled on the mint as we passed it around. We noticed the square stems—a mint family trait—felt the wrinkly, soft leaves, and tasted the small tubular purple flowers. As with garlic, citrus, and hot peppers, strong-flavored herbs like mint provide another example of the way we primates have adapted to enjoy plant compounds that were originally produced as repellants to insects and other predators. Because they are powerful, they may influence us systemically—in other words, they may be medicinal. Mint is no exception, and the effect it had on us was noticeable. It felt cooling, calming, and mildly invigorating, sort of like the feeling of watching gamboling baby goats!

That day, it took no time at all to pick big bunches of fragrant mint to make tea, to send back to the camp kitchens, and to dry for later use. Mint has lots of well-known culinary uses. Try some finely chopped fresh or crushed dried mint in fruit salads, with green peas, and in chocolate cake or brownies. Mint jelly is classically served with rich meats, and mint candies follow a feast to aid digestion and freshen breath.

It Takes One to Know One

Invasives are not easy to love. No matter how beneficial their individual qualities may be, their placement makes their very existence problematic. Now they are here, and no matter how vigorously and aggressively they may be attacked, they cannot be eradicated. Also, many of the methods used against them are extremely problematic in themselves. Their presence is the result of complex, contradictory, and ambiguous forces over which they had no control, but because of the advantages they have due to their function as invaders—an affinity for the climate, a lack of predators and diseases, carrying pests and plagues that weaken local competition—the real problem with invasives is that they come to dominate the landscape, diminishing the resilience and diversity that was natural to the original ecosystem.

The above paragraph could describe a number of invasive plants, such as Japanese knotweed, kudzu, thistle, garlic mustard, bittersweet, and phragmites. It could also describe my colonial ancestors, and, quite frankly, the human species in general. Thus, when we deal with invasive plants, it's a good idea to keep a mirror handy.

The man known as Johnny Appleseed (1774–1845) was a pioneer who "prepared the ground" for the settlers coming after him. He believed in the coming of a New Jerusalem, carried no weapons, and read to his hosts from the Bible and the works of Swedenborg. He was generally well liked. In a series of seasonal moves west, he would plant seeds and then sell the saplings and seedlings to finance his next move. Along with apples, he propagated herbs used as medicines in Europe, including mullein, catnip, horehound, pennyroyal, and fennel. All have proved to be invasive in at least some of the areas in which he planted them. When he died, he was memorialized on the Senate floor as follows: "Your labor has been a labor of love, and generations yet unborn will rise up and call you blessed."[3] Yet

3. Bill Federer, "The Apple & Johnny Appleseed - American Minute with Bill Federer," *American Minute*, March 18, 2021, https://americanminute.com/blogs/todays-american-minute/the-apple-johnny-appleseed-american-minute-with-bill-federer.

despite John's love, humble spirituality, peacefulness, lack of greed, and good intentions, many people have cursed the stinking dog fennel he planted prolifically so as to be available for the treatment of malaria, one of many diseases that came with the settlers.

What to do with invasive plants? Use them if you can. What to do if you are part of an invasive culture, or affected by one? Make yourself useful, and place the health and survival of the natural ecosystems and indigenous cultures of your region, and the world, first and foremost. This can be a difficult shift and a bitter lesson for some of us, who may have been raised with unrealistic expectations, but the study of plants, especially the non-native plants, can be of help.

Observe the knotweed, all of which is clonal—in other words, it is one giant plant spread out into colonies. It has been moved around the world not by seeds, but by bits of stem or root. I remember when it first came to the island; the first place it grew was around telephone poles. Bits of root had been transported to the island on the drilling equipment of the state's highway department. Be careful when you harvest it, and wash your shovel afterward, because it's nearly impossible to eradicate once it gets a toehold. Be careful also because this plant is often unsuitable for use as food or medicine due to "treatment" with toxic herbicides. If you can find a clean patch and are strong and energetic, the root has high concentrations of resveratrol (also found in red wine and grapes) and is tonic to the immune system. If you are less energetic, the spring shoots provide a substantial spring vegetable and can be frozen or put up as chutney, jam, pie filling, and so on. In addition, herbalists have noticed that the spread of knotweed through the eastern United States has correlated rather precisely with the spread of tick-borne Lyme disease, for which the roots of knotweed are a specific medicine. None of us, not even knotweed, are all bad or all good, and the relations between things are more complex than we can fully understand or fairly judge by considering our perspective alone.

Here's another case of setting one invasive species to deal with another. When we bring our goats to conservation land to eat invasive oriental bittersweet, all three of us are invasives on that land. The goats keep the bittersweet from spreading, but they don't completely kill it, and if they did, birds would quickly reseed the area. We're unable to return the land (or ourselves) to any past time or previous state, but we try to strike a new balance, one that increases the abilities of native ecosystems to prevail in at least some areas.

Be aware when harvesting native species that even though they are on home ground and may have been used traditionally, they may well be under some very nontraditional threats and pressures. Between clearing, paving and building, competition from invasive competitors, and strange new diseases, they may need some encouragement. If they are rare, discover alternatives, refrain from harvesting, and, if possible, learn to grow and spread them. United Plant

Savers is an organization that can help with this.[4] The best foragers today focus on using invasive plants and harvesting them in ways that leave more room for rare natives. Some do a "reverse Johnny Appleseed" maneuver and plant garden-grown native seeds and roots where they have dug invasive roots.

I have been hesitant to write about foraging because of worries that increased foraging may further threaten native ecosystems. Even being common is not enough protection; think of the Atlantic sturgeon, the American chestnut, or the passenger pigeon—all abundant, delicious, and fortifying staples in their day, but now endangered or extinct. On the other hand, I believe that people's perceived disconnect from our surroundings is part of the problem, and that foraging can be a useful antidote, since we naturally tend to notice available food. The answer to this puzzle comes from invasive plants; by eating and using them, we can bring the system toward rather than away from a desirable dynamic balance. To help the larger systems of which we are a part move closer to balance is an honor, and to do so by finding and eating delicious food is a win-win. The real benefit to us, besides the goodies, is the noticing and nature connection. When we perceive ourselves as dominating from the top of some food pyramid or chain, our actions cannot help but miss the mark and become destructive, because they are based on lies and

4. Contact information for United Plant Savers: United Plant Savers, PO Box 147, Rutland, OH 45775, (740) 742-3455, office@UnitedPlantSavers.org.

false premises. Connection and awareness allow us to act more realistically and effectively within our environment as part of a web of complex interrelationships, which include our food choices.

Some plants from Africa, Asia, Europe, and elsewhere have moved to the Americas, and vice versa, without behaving invasively. They changed the patterns, but did not disrupt them entirely, the way invasives do. They became one of many—common, but not exclusive. Such plants, including clover, plantain, and many more, can help guide us as we continue to explore, develop, repair, and improve our vital relationship with the biosphere—the external world—and one another.

Plant Portrait: Garlic Mustard
(Alliaria petiolata)

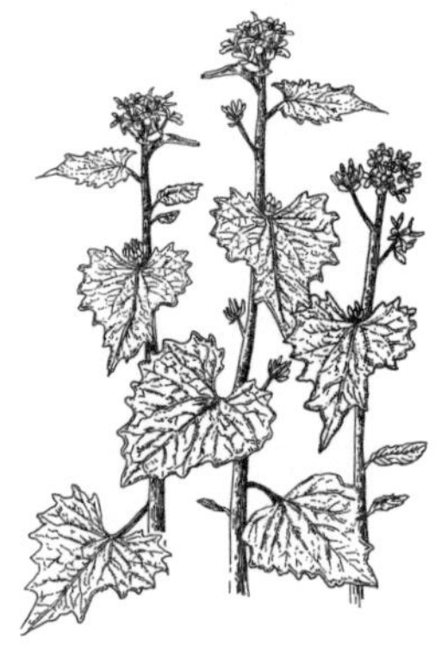

Garlic mustard is a useful and delicious plant. All of it is edible. As indicated by the name, it provides familiar flavors and medicinal attributes. It is one of the earliest greens in spring, starting as a low rosette of dark green, scalloped, crinkled leaves with a distinctive garlicky scent and flavor (they make excellent leaf crisps). There's quite a long harvest window before the leaves get rank and bitter as the plant begins to bloom. Then, the buds and lacy white flowers are good for decorating savory dishes. The seeds, like mustard seeds, can be coarsely crushed or finely ground, moistened with a little water or vinegar, and used as a condiment. The roots taste like mild, garlicky horseradish and can be used similarly. Try them in tartar sauce or deviled eggs, as a stir-fry ingredient, or in pickles.

Garlic mustard is not an old friend from childhood, but a new arrival. The first time I saw it growing by the side of the road, I thought, *What's that pretty white flower that I don't recognize?* Next, it popped up by the compost heap, and nowadays I try to harvest it before it goes to seed whenever possible, to slow its spread. Why not welcome such a tasty new neighbor? Garlic mustard is very invasive, meaning it takes over. The roots exude compounds that kill other plants growing near it and prevent their seeds from sprouting, and it has quickly overrun large areas of previously diverse forest understory. This makes it an excellent candidate for large-scale harvesting and for inclusion in products made in bulk. However, don't eat huge quantities of the very young leaves at one time, as they can contain traces of the toxins that help make this plant so invasive.

Invasive Recipes

Invasive plants are excellent targets for foragers. Your state has an official list of plants considered invasive in your region. Just make sure to harvest from an area that has not been treated with herbicides. Invasives provide an exception to the harvesting rule of take a little, leave a lot. Unlike noninvasive and native foraged foods, as long as you have the landowner's permission, it is acceptable to pick them all, if you can. Most likely, you will not be able to eliminate them, but you will develop favorite patches and seasons for harvest, and perhaps you can slow their advance, especially if you repeatedly clear out an area. Be cautious with disposal of seeds and roots so you do not inadvertently spread them. Don't be rude or hateful, however. Each plant has a reason for being where they are. Many weeds thrive in what biologists call disturbed soil … and who disturbed the soil?

If you want to feed the hungry, educate the public, and spread the knowledge of foraging, focusing on the invasive plants in your area will ensure that you are contributing your love and knowledge toward effective actions with environmental benefits and helping to right the balance of nature. Since the natural tendencies of ecosystems usually lean toward coming into balance or equilibrium, when we are engaged in this work, we may feel the power and support of much larger evolutionary forces than those concerned with small-scale individual survival. It's even possible that this environmental propriety and correctness can make our harvests taste better. Try it and see what you think.

Recipe: Mother's Mint Jelly

- 3½ cups of apple juice (crab apple or Granny Smith is preferred, but frozen will do well also)
- 1½ cups of strong mint infusion (fill a heatproof container loosely with fresh mint, cover with water just about to boil, cover and steep for five minutes, then strain)
- 6½ cups of sugar
- 1 box of pectin
- 5 drops of green food coloring (optional, but without it, the jelly will be straw-colored)

This method may be used to make any kind of herb jelly. To make the jelly, follow the directions for "apple" on the box of pectin, replacing the water with your herbal infusion.

Recipe: Knotweed Marmalade or Conserve

- 6 generous cups of Japanese knotweed, diced small (about 2 pounds, or use a combination of knotweed and rhubarb)
- 6 cups of sugar
- 4 oranges, grated rinds and juice
- 2 lemons, grated rinds and juice
- 1 cinnamon stick

Cook all together carefully on low for about one hour, stirring often. Remove cinnamon stick. To make this into a conserve, add a half pound of chopped almonds and/or dark or golden raisins to the hot mixture after cooking. Packed hot into hot jars, this relish will keep a month or more in the fridge, or you may can it for ten minutes in a hot water bath to sterilize and seal it for long-term storage.

Recipe: Horehound Cough Drops

- About 2 cups of fresh horehound leaves
- 1 cup of granulated sugar
- ½ cup of honey (it does not need to be raw honey as it will be boiled)

Candy making is best done in dry weather. Pick a time when you can focus without interruptions; candy making is demanding, and sugar syrup is flammable and can cause dangerous burns. A candy thermometer is recommended.

Make a strong tea as a base. Place crumpled and crushed horehound tips in a pan with a tight-fitting lid. Barely cover the tips with water, bring to a simmer, cover, and let steep for fifteen minutes or so. Strain and measure out one cup of strong tea. If you feel it is not strong enough, repeat the process, pouring the tea over fresh leaves. It should be quite bitter.

Lay out small candy molds on a heatproof, rimmed baking pan. Silicone molds are the easiest to use. If you have no molds, it is possible to make your own using a shallow baking pan half filled with confectioners' sugar. Make dents and dimples in the sugar and pour the candy into them. Although just as tasty and effective as molded drops, they will be spiky and uneven in shape and size. My mother's method was to pour and spread the candy out thinly on a piece of buttered parchment paper set in a rimmed pan.

After the candy has hardened, it can be shattered into pieces like brittle. The disadvantage of this method is that you end up with a lot of candy dust and irregularly sized and very sharp pieces, which must be licked with care at first, but they still work to quell a cough.

To cook the candy, combine one cup of the strong tea with the sugar and honey in a large, heavy-bottomed pot over medium-high heat. Add the candy thermometer and stir until the sugar has dissolved. There is a technique to stirring the candy: you want to stir up the bottom while avoiding the sides of the pan. If you stir in crystals from the sides of the pan, the whole batch may crystallize before you are ready. When the temperature on the thermometer goes over 250 degrees Fahrenheit, you will need to stir constantly, still avoiding the sides. When it reaches 300 degrees Fahrenheit, carefully pour into the prepared molds. Cool several hours or overnight. Toss with confectioners' sugar or cornstarch and store in an airtight container at room temperature. It's helpful to layer wax or parchment paper between the candies so they don't stick together.

This temperature is for hard candies. If you like them soft, sticky, and chewy, like toffee, aim for about 280 degrees Fahrenheit.

Before candy thermometers were widely available, the way to test candy syrup was to drop a small spoonful into ice water. This gives a quick analysis of how hard the candy will be when cooled. The soft crack stage is between 270 and 290 degrees Fahrenheit, while temperatures of 295 degrees Fahrenheit and up have reached the hard crack stage. This method takes some practice; if your experiments don't come out the way you had hoped, you can always melt them down with a little water or lemon juice and use them for cough syrup.

This recipe can be used with any flavored liquid as the base—ginger lemon, for example, is very good.

Recipe: Coleslaw

Leaves that may be a bit strong on their own, such as violet, yellow dock, or garlic mustard, finely shredded, make an excellent addition to mayonnaise-based dishes like macaroni, potato, or egg salads. Try a coleslaw made with regular cabbage combined with some shredded wild dark green leaves, grated carrots, radishes, or other colorful vegetables and some spring onion greens. Garnish with early flowers like violets, primroses, or chickweed for a dish that deliciously defines the transition from winter to spring.

Recipe: To Dry Herbs

In the morning, after the dew has dried, pick a large bunch of your chosen herb and hang it upside down in a paper bag. You may tie a string or put a rubber band around the neck of the bag to keep out dust. Label the bag with the species and date. Hang it in a dry, airy place until the herbs are dry and crisp, then store in a labeled, airtight, and lightproof container in a cool spot. For tea, use stems and all; for cooking, use just the leaves, stored whole and crumbled as needed.

Beverage: Mint Tea

Mint is full of volatile compounds. This is evident because it's strongly flavored and easily releases a distinctive scent—the aroma is molecules leaving the plant material and diffusing into the air. When dried leaves have little or no scent, they will have little or no flavor, and should be replaced. Fragrant herbs require gentle handling—boiling or steeping them too long brings out their less delicate flavors. Make mint tea with water that has come off the boil (about 190 degrees Fahrenheit) and pour the tea off the leaves after two or three minutes. Alternatively, use the cold infusion method, leaving mint sprigs in cold water in the fridge overnight. Mint makes excellent sun tea, too. Depending on how strong you want it, use one small sprig of mint for each cup or two of water.

Occasionally, someone taking homeopathic remedies will be advised to avoid mint, so be sure that everyone is aware if you include it in mixtures. Its stomach-settling attributes, and the way it energizes without stimulating, makes it a popular tea for children, elders, and convalescents, and its vigorous taste can be used in blends to enhance or mask medicinal flavors. The mint family is large and diverse; usually lemon balm, spearmint, and peppermint are favored for teas, but feel free to experiment.

Practice: Observing Biodiversity and Monoculture

This interesting practice doesn't require *doing* anything. It is strictly a noticing exercise. It asks that you observe feelings and reactions in yourself and others, including plants and animals, in environments with differing levels of diversity. How many species surround you? How many languages? What is missing? What sorts of contrast or sameness can you notice? Which things would you prefer to see "broken up," and which would you wish to smooth out and make more even? Notice the difference between an old-growth forest and a tree farm with trees of the same species and age planted in rows. How do you feel looking at a picture of people dressed alike compared to the same people in varied styles of clothing? What are the differences between a random cluster and a regular grid? Do your best to suspend judgment. This is not a "good or bad" evaluation, because such dichotomies are far too simplistic to explain the complexity of nature, and much depends on our perspective. A rainforest or ocean may appear very diverse at close range, and completely uniform from space, while cloud patterns may be the opposite. Part of the value of this exercise is the insight it can provide into our own reactions and the reasons for them. Where are we most comfortable? What level of complexity makes us feel at home? Under what conditions do we do our best work? What is beautiful? A greater understanding of the effects of diversity and monoculture is useful as we plan future endeavors, design spaces, and organize projects.

List: Some Edible Invasive Plants

Here is a short, incomplete list of plants that the National Audubon Society considers invasive in Massachusetts and that have edible parts. Keep in mind that these plants are relatively new to us, and we are still learning about how they behave here—in the environment, as medicine, and in the kitchen—so it's always a good idea to look into the ways they are used in their native lands.

wineberry	*Rubus phoenicolasius*	berries, leaves as tea
wild chervil	*Anthriscus sylvestris*	use with caution, toxic look-alikes
pepperweed	*Lepidium virginicum*	all parts in season
multiflora rose	*Rosa multiflora*	flowers, hips
Japanese knotweed	*Fallopia japonica*	young shoots, roots as medicine
Japanese honeysuckle	*Lonicera japonica*	flowers only
bush honeysuckles	*Lonicera* spp.	flowers only
hardy kiwi	*Actinidia arguta*	fruit
garlic mustard	*Alliaria petiolata*	all parts in season
dame's rocket	*Hesperis matronalis*	early leaves, buds, flowers
barberry	*Berberis vulgaris, thunbergii*	fruit
black locust	*Robinia pseudoacacia*	flowers
kudzu	*Pueraria montana*	leaves, shoots, flowers, roots
autumn olive	*Elaeagnus umbellata*	fruit
common reed	*Phragmites australis*	young shoots, gum

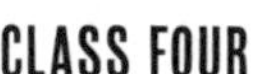

Finding Corresponding Flavors

Most foragers like to try new foods, and some have highly developed palates. Others would like to recreate favorite dishes using local ingredients. Still others simply enjoy exploring new tastes and techniques out of curiosity. Here are some ideas for ingredient conversions, using the flavor of lemons as an example, and for expanding on methods, with pesto making as an example. Finally, there are "blank canvas" recipes to test new flavors and combinations, and an exercise routine for your taste buds. These explorations are great for expanding your awareness of flavors and how they work, eventually allowing you to develop your own personal favorite recipes using what grows around you.

When Life Does Not Give You Lemons

Foraged foods can provide new flavors and expand the range of herbs and spices available to the adventurous cook. It's ironic that most of us are familiar with exotic tropical spices like cinnamon and black pepper in the kitchen, although we might not recognize the plants that they came from. Meanwhile, equally dynamic flavors may be growing all around us unremarked. Those who have explored the possibilities of their regional flavorings often come to the opinion that dishes made from entirely local ingredients have an easy coherence and integrity that is tangibly satisfying. Certainly, when one is consciously working with a specific piece of land, the spirits of place, or the connection with local history, dishes cooked entirely from the territory concerned have great power and focus and are an important component of sacred and ancestral food offerings in many traditions.

Locally foraged ingredients are fresh and have (hopefully) not been sprayed or irradiated. A person attentively harvesting, processing, and storing plant materials in relatively small amounts for personal and household use can quite easily surpass the quality of the best (and most expensive) commercial products. Little or no cost is involved—instead of money, the investment here is in time, knowledge, and care.

Eventually, experimentation will lead to the development of local specialties and personal favorites. As long as the experimentation stays within the realm of known edibles, there is no "wrong" if the results taste good. However, to get started, it is helpful to make comparisons to flavors that are already familiar. Since not many cookbooks mention foraged flavors, such comparisons are also helpful in the adaptation of recipes.

For example, there are quite a few plants with a flavor reminiscent of lemons. Most probably contain vitamin C, whose acidic tartness is familiar and appealing. None of them taste exactly like lemons, but the ways we use lemons can provide inspiration for working with them: in a sweet and sour summer drink, in salad dressings, with fish, or to enhance rich and creamy desserts. Quantities, materials, and preparation methods may need alteration, but favorite recipes and combinations are a good place to start for those wishing to develop their own local versions of classic dishes.

Sadly, lemons don't grow on Martha's Vineyard, but here are some of my favorite foraged "lemony" herbs:

- **GRAPE LEAVES:** As discussed in the chapter on cooking techniques, grape leaves impart a mild lemon flavor to whatever is wrapped in them.
- **CATBRIER TENDRILS:** In spring, these gorgeously beautiful shining red curls are sour and somewhat acrid, great for garnish and outdoor nibbling.

- **BLUEBERRY FLOWERS:** Try not to eat too many, since they are potential berries!
- **SHEEP SORREL:** Wild sorrel is a pest of flowerbeds—it's well worth eating what you weed out, especially in the spring and fall.
- **OXALIS:** Delicate, clover-shaped leaves and yellow flowers pack a lemony punch; a few in a salad will make it taste "dressed."
- **LEMON BALM:** A garden escape, lemon balm naturalizes here, but not invasively. It makes a great tea, with a mild lemon and mint taste that most people love.
- **SUMAC:** The red berries make a lovely pink "ade" that can substitute for lemon juice.
- **HIBISCUS FLOWERS:** Fresh or dried, they add color, flavor, and vitamin C to cold drinks and hot tea (called sorrel in the Caribbean).
- **LEMONGRASS, LEMON MYRTLE, AND LEMON VERBENA:** These can be grown from seeds or slips in the garden in summer and taken in as striking, delicious, and fragrant houseplants in winter.
- **LEMON AND LIME:** Citrus seeds may be sprouted and grown in pots. You will probably not have enough sun to get fruit, but the fresh leaves are a prized seasoning.

Without being precisely lemony, vinegars and pickling brines, yogurt, wine, and other products of fermentation may add sour notes to your flavor profile. Also consider unripe fruits such as green grapes or crab apples. Finally, our most lemony local fruit, the cranberry, dries, freezes, and preserves well, and it is a powerhouse of nutrition, especially in winter.

When a standard recipe calls for lemon, consider whether any of the above flavors would also go well. Perhaps a "lemon herb" tincture could replace extract, or a lemony tea could sub out for water, or a sprinkling of tart flowers could go over the top. You may end up creating a new treat, one you look forward to every year as its season arrives.

Similar comparisons and associations may be made for other favorite flavors. Here are a few more examples:

- **PEPPER AND MUSTARD:** Seeds, greens, and flowers from the large and abundant wild mustard clan; also, those of wild radishes, shepherd's purse, peppergrass, cresses, and nasturtiums.
- **ONION AND GARLIC:** Wild leeks and chives, ramps, garlic mustard.
- **WARM SPICES:** Carolina allspice, sassafras, sweet pepperbush, bayberry.
- **AROMATICS:** Pine needles and spruce tips, sap, juniper berries, yarrow, wintergreen.

Adapting Techniques

As with flavorings, techniques used in traditional recipes may provide inspiration for ways to use foraged ingredients. For example, the Italian sauce, pesto, is made with basil, olive oil, garlic, pine nuts, and parmesan cheese, pounded together by hand. Originally used to finish soups, pesto has spread far beyond its roots and nowadays is used in lots of creative ways.

The recipe can be adopted and adapted to other herbs than basil, other nuts than pine, even other oils than olive. The mortar and pestle may be replaced by a food processor, and the product may be frozen, so the texture will be different. The goal is not to imitate pesto, or to create something "mock" that people will mistake for the real thing. Instead, local ingredients combine to make something fresh and new, unique to the time, place, and people that have brought it forth. The result is no longer pesto, but a delicious pesto-inspired sauce that can be used in similar ways.

Deconstructing further, we find that what really preserves the basil's fresh taste is being pulverized in oil. Any foraged herbs and flowers, singly or combined, can be pounded, blended, or processed with any oil or grease and refrigerated or frozen. This method preserves fresh flavor, raw nutrition, and vivifying color for long-term storage. And while the flavors will be very different from those of basil, pine nuts, and olives, we still know how to use our new creations—like pesto.

A closely related product is herb butter. Its uses are almost endless, but it is probably best known for adding a fresh and savory finishing touch to a wide variety of foods, from soups and sauces to steamed vegetables, grains, meats, and seafood. Similar compounds can be made with any kind of grease, such as poultry fat, lard, nut butter, coconut oil, and so on.

Plant Portrait: Sumac
(Rhus spp.)

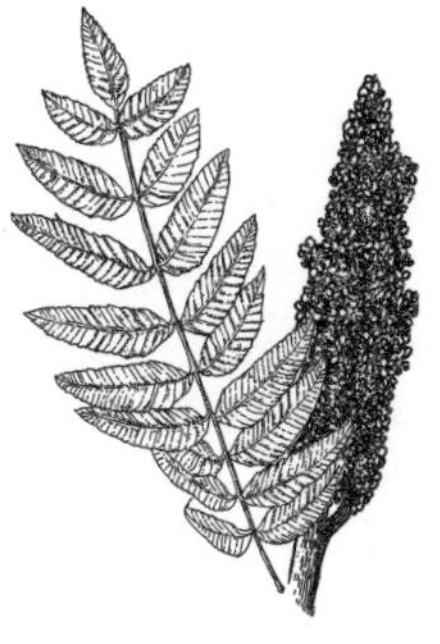

Sumac is considered an invasive weed in some places because it can grow under hot, dry, less-than-fertile conditions. Sumac's shiny, regular leaves and upright seed clusters are attractive, and it won't get bigger than a small tree or large bush. It is often planted along highways for erosion control. While it is not desirable to harvest near busy roads because of contaminants from exhaust and runoff, the roadside populations can alert you when Sumac is ready to pick in a less polluted area.

Sometimes it is not possible to access clean land to harvest from. This is a personal call, but in this case, I will harvest wherever I am; if

I am in a toxic environment with an adaptable plant, we may as well help each other, if we can. The plants can help heal and feed us and even help clean the air and soil, but it is up to us to stop the spread of our own toxicity. Plants can't do that.

There are several different kinds of sumac, and all are edible, except one: poison sumac. Poison sumac is not a true sumac; it comes from a different plant family—it is in fact a close relative of poison ivy, and it will give you a nasty rash if you touch it. Its habit of growth and compound leaves are similar to the true sumacs, but the berries of poison sumac are dead white, while edible sumacs have red berries, even when immature. Poison sumac is uncommon in our region and mostly grows in swamps. If you encounter it, give it a wide berth.

Once you see red seed clusters, you know you have one of the edible varieties—staghorn sumac is the most common. It is interesting to watch the spikes or clusters of seeds ripening and to evaluate the optimum harvest time with an eye to the weather. Examined closely, the seeds are covered with small shiny resinous hairs that break off and stick to your fingers—these hairs are where the flavor develops as the seeds ripen. Because the clusters are water soluble, long hard rains will weaken the flavor considerably. Try to sample frequently and harvest briskly, especially if rainy weather is predicted. Handling will knock off the tasty hairs, so use a gentle touch and break up the seed clusters just enough to spread out and dry until crisp without stirring or rubbing. Store away from heat, light, and air. Sumac is used as a seasoning in North Africa and the Middle East, where it's combined with salt, toasted sesame seeds, wild oregano, thyme, hyssop, or other herbs to create Za'atar, a traditional spice mix used in cooking and as a dip with olive oil.

Blank Canvas Recipes for Culinary Explorations

The following blank canvas recipes, made in tiny quantities, provide tools for testing new flavors and experimenting with blends. Just replace "one cup" with "one tablespoon" for a sample-sized batch. Once you have developed a version that you like, larger quantities can be made to provide kitchen and pantry staples with a flavorful twist. They are excellent gifts for foodies and allow those of us who can forage only occasionally a way to prolong the enjoyment from a fruitful expedition. Every year these recipes extend past frost and into the colder months, when a taste of summer's colors and flavors can go a long way to remind us of the bounty that surrounds us.

Recipe: Herb or Flower Butter

- 1 cup of flowers, petals only, or ¼ to ½ cup of aromatic herbs, or a combination
- 1 cup of butter, softened

Finely chop plant materials, mix with butter, and let stand covered at room temperature for two or three hours. Roll in parchment or waxed paper to form a log, and refrigerate or freeze for up to six months. Slices may be cut off the log as needed, and the rest returned to the freezer. Use flavored butters for finishing roasted and grilled foods, to spread on biscuits, or in an elegant pound cake.

Recipe: Herb or Flower Sugar

- ½ cup of chopped sweet flowers and/or aromatic herbs like spruce tips or mint
- 2 cups of granulated sugar

Pulverize sugar and plant materials in a mortar or food processor. Store in a clean jar for one week, sift, and store airtight. Sprinkle on fruit, make sugar cookies, or serve with tea.

Recipe: Herb or Flower Salt

Finely chop plant materials (or blend in a food processor) and mix with plenty of salt—roughly ¾ plant to ¼ salt, but proportions do not need to be precise. Packed into a clean jar and stored in the fridge, this salty paste will keep indefinitely, and can be used, measure for measure, in place of plain salt. It can really elevate a winter soup or a pot of beans.

Recipe: Herb or Flower Alcohol

To experiment with flavor, a relatively neutral base, like vodka, is recommended, but any alcohol will draw out flavors and active compounds. Rum was typically used during the island's seafaring, whaling, and slaving eras, and can be useful for lineage healing work. Traditional European blends often use brandy and feature plants known for medicine as well as flavor. A strong alcohol extraction is called a tincture in medicine making, and an extract in the kitchen. Only a few drops are needed. A less concentrated extraction can be used for mixed drinks and cordials, to muddle fruit, or in desserts. Experiment with adding more or less plant material to your base until the desired strength is reached. Steep for one month or more; straining is optional. Choose a glass container and put in your plant material according to strength desired. Some strong-flavored extracts like vanilla require only a couple of beans, others such as the herbs usually take more, but not more than three quarters full and loosely packed, so that the plant materials can swim around. Fill the container almost to the brim and cover tightly so the alcohol doesn't evaporate.

Recipe: Herb or Flower Oil

Loosely fill a container three-fourths full with plant material. Avoid large chunks, which could mold. Remove petals from large flower centers or leaves from thick stems. If the material is very juicy, let it wilt in a shady, airy place until it has lost weight and volume. Cover with cooking oil. Steep for one month in the fridge. To use, strain and rebottle, or just pour the oil off the top as needed.

Recipe: Herb or Flower Vinegar

Place wilted or dried plant materials in a clean bottle or jar—anywhere from a sprig or two up to three-fourths full. Fresh plants may be used but have a tendency to mold. Cover with vinegar of choice, and steep for one month. Straining is optional. For gifts, strain into an ornamental bottle with a fresh sprig or blossom and tie a ribbon around the neck. Flavored vinegars shine in salad dressings and marinades and as exotic drizzles.

SOLAR AND LUNAR EXTRACTIONS:

I have given instructions for lunar extractions, which use time to draw out the essence of the plant materials. One month, or one lunar cycle, is the minimum—longer is fine, too. However, if you are in a hurry, you may use heat to release the flavor; this is a solar extraction. This faster technique is for oil or vinegar only—do NOT heat alcohol! Take your container of plants and liquid and place it in a pan of water and heat very gently and slowly to just below a simmer. Don't allow it to boil. Remove the whole pan from the heat and let your potion stand in the water overnight, cooling slowly. This replaces the one-month steeping period. The solar method is also used when making herbal honeys.

Beverage: Sumac-ade

The taste of sumac is sour, reminiscent of lemon juice. That sour, citrusy flavor tells the tongue that vitamin C is present, especially when raw and fresh. When developing recipes with foraged ingredients, sumac seeds can add flavor and crunch along with lemony flavor. To lose the crunch, steep the seeds in liquid, stir, and strain. The liquid may be hot, as for tea, but the best flavor comes from steeping the seeds in cold water. Cold brewing extracts the flavors while stored overnight (or up to three days) in the fridge. This method is especially nice with berries; besides sumac, tossing a few straw-, wine-, black-, or blueberries in a quart of water makes a very refreshing summer drink. Mint also extracts well using cold brewing, and it's a good method to try anytime. Hot infusions bring out flavors that are too strong or tend to become rank or bitter. Use a handful or more of sumac berries, fresh or dried, per gallon of water, or to taste. The resulting sour, pink liquid may be used to make sumac "pink lemonade." Dilute if necessary and add honey or any sweetener of choice. This pretty and refreshing drink was a beloved feature of our summer childhoods, garnished with a mint leaf or a colorful, honey-flavored flower. Sumac-ade is also good in mixed drinks, in a shandy, or as a component of herbal sodas or beers. In the field, sucking on ripe red sumac seeds will make you pucker, give you a flavorful burst of vitamin C, and help stave off thirst. Try dropping a small cluster into your water bottle!

Practice: Flavor Tester

Like any other skill, taste buds can refine their ability to distinguish the fine points of flavor through repetition and practice. Part of the process of adaptation consists of developing the ability to see (or taste) the widest possible range of options. This technique allows you to explore and expand your palate, and to get to know a chosen ingredient intimately. Some plant flavors extract in oil and not in water, and vice versa, and the volatile substances can be diminished or altered by heat as well, so you will get different flavor ranges, colors, and aromas depending how you prepare the material. Try this easy experiment with a new herb or one that's familiar—you might be surprised at the range of possibilities.

1. Make sure you have identified your plant and that it is edible.
2. Try a little nibble—if it is a seasoning herb, it will probably be rather strong to eat plain.

3. Boil two cups of water in a saucepan.
4. Place a few leaves in a cup and cover with half the hot water as if making tea.
5. Simmer a few more leaves in the rest of the water as if making soup.
6. Chop a few more leaves with butter, grease, or oil of your choice.
7. Spread half of the butter, grease, or oil mixture on bread or crackers.
8. Use the other half to sauté something bland like egg, cooked rice, or noodles.

This technique provides the opportunity to try the flavors contained in the herb five ways: plain and raw, in a low heat water extraction, in a boiling water extraction, as a raw oil-based compound, and as a cooked oil-based compound. The entire experiment can be performed in fifteen minutes, snack included.

This exercise, and experiments in general, make clear to us and to the rest of the cosmos that our reality is not permanently fixed, predetermined, or without question. The ability to adapt—whether for a cook updating a family recipe, a farmer breeding the tastiest version of a vegetable variety, or a species adapting to evolutionary pressure—requires the admission that things can be, and perhaps should be, very different. It requires that we be honest about what options are available, and about what will actually work. Although tasting a new plant you have prepared in several ways is a relatively minor form of alchemy, it models the type of exploratory, creative, responsive perception that prepares the ground for healing change, drives off inertia, and opens new paths for further experiments.

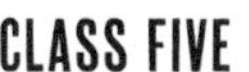

CLASS FIVE

Eating Flowers

Flowers are some of the most easily recognizable plant parts. They are generally easier to tell apart than roots, seeds, leaves, or even berries. Although they do not store well, nor are they likely to stave off real hunger, in their season, they provide us with such an abundance of delightful colors, scents, and flavors that they always seem like a special kind of gift. There is a partial list of edible flowers at the end of this book. Sadly, it's not a good idea to eat flowers from the florist—they are often treated with pesticides and inedible chemicals to make them last longer. It's much better to pick your own … and because freshness is so important when serving flowers and they make such a dramatic statement, they can really make the forager shine!

Flowers and the Gift Economy

Flowers are magical expressions of beauty and desire, and many of them are extremely tasty. Not all flowers are edible, even those from plants with other edible parts—it is not recommended to eat potato or tomato flowers, for example. Don't eat crocuses or daffodils! Tulips, however, are lovely stuffed with a filling of your choice. (I like cheese fillings, but herbed rice or other grains, egg salad, and even sweet spreads go well, also.) Most food plants have flowers that taste like the plant they came from—radishes and arugula taste spicy; borage flowers taste like cucumber. Others have their own unique tastes. Once you know a family of plants has edible flowers, sample and form your own opinions and preferences. Some people find nasturtium flowers too hot; others love the spicy salsa taste and discover that each color has a slightly different flavor. Once you become familiar with the range of flavors you are working with, you can decide how best to use them to complement your cooking. You might not want to add nasturtiums to a sweet and mild fruit salad, but they are fabulous and dramatic on tacos, or to garnish bland cheese, or on a sandwich instead of mustard.

There are flowers to be found throughout the growing season. In the spring, violets and primroses add color and tonic vitamins to the first green salads, along with starry chickweed. Later, mullein and evening primrose offer mild, substantial, butter-yellow flowers that can be picked and repicked, since new ones open daily. Many garden vegetables like squash and beans provide bonus flower harvests in addition to their main crop. Flowers have great decorative potential, adding color and interest both as ingredients and garnishes. Many are nutritional and medicinal powerhouses. Unwilted flowers indicate a dewy freshness and a proximity to the sources of abundance, whether garden, forest, or field. Although at their best fresh, if carefully dried, candied, or otherwise preserved, they can bring joy, color, and a taste of spring sunshine to midwinter days.

While in the field, you don't have to be a kid to enjoy the nectar from invasive but beautiful silver- and gold-flowered honeysuckle. If you know a child who hasn't been introduced to the pleasures of "honeysuckers," do your duty, and pass it on! Show them the viny habit, the two-sided leaf—shiny above and velvety below—and the two colors of flowers right next to each other ... then show them how to pick a flower, bite off the base, and drink sweet nectar like a bee.

Speaking of bees, we remember that the purpose of flowers, with their extravagant shapes, colors, scents, and tastes, is to attract pollinators: bees of many kinds, moths, other insects, even hummingbirds. Their beauty in our eyes is extra—not necessary to the main purpose, a gift. Maybe that's why flowers have always been favored as gifts and offerings, full of sentimental meaning. Gifts—beauty above and beyond what is necessary—are found abundantly in nature, and our gratitude and capacity for appreciation, noticing, and receptivity are essential components of the creation process. Without recipients, one cannot give gifts, and without a perceiver, beauty would not exist. Although there is an exchange taking place, gifts such as floral beauty are not transactions, not even with the bee. One reason bees are so sensitive to pesticides and pollution is that—unlike leaf eaters like ourselves, who are used to being chemically repulsed and adapt rapidly—bees have generally been welcomed by flowers and have not evolved to process poisons.

Gifts require attention and participation, and they carry a certain obligation to amplify or create beauty. The fertile effectiveness of creative collaboration and mutual inspiration is evident in a patch of flowers buzzing with insects, and also in the activities of Camp Jabberwocky, as anyone who has been lucky enough to attend one of their zany musical plays can attest. The importance of pollination, both literal and figurative, cannot be overstated. Gifts multiply, flowers bear fruit, and beauty ripples outward like the hum of bees.

There is a place at Camp Jabberwocky, on one of the lower trails, where in early summer a scattering of fragile white petals may decorate the path, especially after a rain. If you happen by on an August morning, it is possible to pick raspberries, blackberries, and highbush blueberries together, and lots of them hang over the paved path where they can be reached from a wheelchair. The berries are happy there, because there is swampland below, and the hollow catches and amplifies the light and heat of the sun. You will perspire while picking, it's impossible to avoid a few bramble scratches, and there are mosquitoes. These slight discomforts, if anything, enhance the taste of extremely ripe berries warmed by the sun and eaten on the spot.

My berry-picking Grandma advised me to eat all I could while picking. She didn't want me getting into her bucket after we got home—those were for the kitchen, to become muffins, pancakes, pies, and jam. She also pointed out, with a wink, that the berries you have eaten cannot be spilled. (I was a clumsy child.) She picked into a coffee can hung round her neck by a string, so that she could use both hands, and in a good season, she would pick enough for a pie or two before breakfast. She always thanked the bushes, which are now more than a century old, and still generous.

Often people approach foraging as a survival technique, a hedge against deprivation, and a way to reduce the grocery bill. There's nothing wrong with that approach, of course, and whenever you may be short of other food, I wish you an abundance of nutritious weeds and the ability to utilize them. However, my own experience of foraging has been more like receiving a series of recurring gifts. Rather than being a product of need, eaten only because there is nothing else, each delicacy I have come to know enriches my everyday experience. I see the buds on the honeysuckle vines, and the delicate white blossoms falling from the berry bushes and brambles, and I anticipate the sweetness that is coming. Honeysuckle and other flowers will not save us from starvation, but they bring joy every year in their season—perhaps they feed a different hunger. Many a poet has compared our fleeting, fading, beautiful lives to those of our favorite flowers.

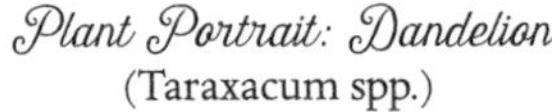

(Taraxacum spp.)

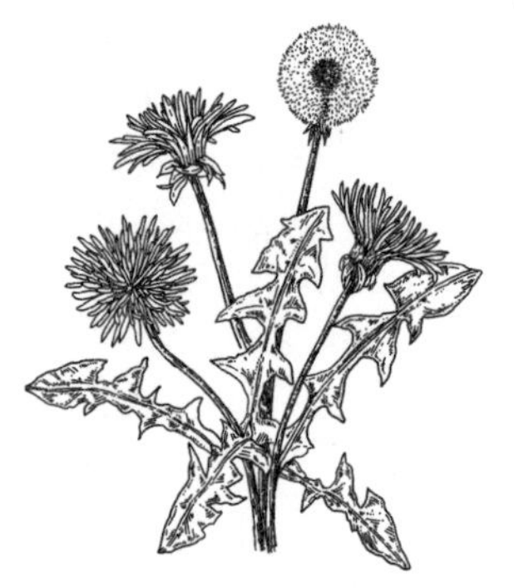

When you say, "Weeds," most Americans think of dandelions. Though regarded as a pest of lawns, in many places, they are valued as culinary and medicinal treasures. However, there's one important thing to consider before setting out to gather them—timing. Most of us first learn to recognize dandelions by the flowers and seed heads, and this is not the time to harvest the leaves… dandelion leaves are mild and tasty until the plant begins to bloom, and they become extremely bitter once flowering begins. Going bitter while flowering is a common plant strategy. It allows for grazing to occur while the plant is young and the expendable young leaves are tender and sweet, which strengthens the plant's root system, and then calls for grazing to cease when the vulnerable aboveground flower stalk begins to emerge. This strategy dictates the forager's harvest schedule for many types of plants besides dandelions: leaves in spring, buds and flowers all summer, seeds and roots in the fall.

Learn to recognize dandelion leaves before the flowers arrive. They are perennial, coming up from the same root year after year, so if you only know them in bloom, take notice of a plant growing near you and follow it through its life cycle to become familiar with it. The leaves are best picked when the power is rising upward from the root toward the spring sun for a traditional cleansing and tonic dish. Once the plants begin to bloom (indicating that the soil has warmed enough to plant potatoes), look for the unopened flower buds, round and firm, that can sometimes be found in clusters on plants in rich soil. Rinse and add to stir-fries or soups, or dip very briefly (one minute) in boiling water, cool, and add to cold dishes. They are extremely tasty and very versatile.

The golden petals plucked from the flowers are dried for tea, made into wine and cordial, used as garnish, and added to dishes for color and a tangy, somewhat bitter flavor. The whole flowers make wonderful fritters. The seeds are bitter and may be used as seasoning. The roots fatten and become starchier and sweeter as the leaves die back and the plants move their energy underground. They are dried for healthful teas, roasted for a dark bitter drink (somewhat resembling coffee but without caffeine), or prepared as a chewy, jerkylike snack. A few fat fall dandelion roots in sandy soil in a bucket will produce a surprising quantity of tender leaves if brought into a warm place in midwinter and watered. Like endive, a relative, they may be eaten green or covered and blanched white. When everything outside is frozen, a few fresh, flavorful, home-foraged leaves are very exciting.

Although the focus here is on food rather than on medicine, I would be remiss if I did not mention that dandelion in all its forms is a cleansing herb that particularly acts on the kidneys. Its French folk name is *pissenlit*, or "wet the bed." It is a diuretic and will make you pee, though hopefully not in bed. Unlike most diuretics, dandelion supplies more potassium (and some other minerals) than it washes out, making it useful for people who have difficulty with water retention. Although its curative powers are legendary, you don't have to feel unwell to enjoy the taste and nutrition of this common and familiar plant. It holds its own as a gourmet vegetable, with a depth of flavor so satisfying that its many admirers eagerly await its emergence every year.

Flower Recipes

Flowers are usually used as garnishes rather than forming the main part of the dish, so even a few can have a big impact. A bouquet of edible flowers makes an interesting and lovely hostess gift, but otherwise, you will not usually need the stems, and can just pluck off the flower heads; this often goes much quicker than picking stem by stem. One concern with flowers is that they may contain small insects such as ants. If I am using large flowers like nasturtiums or squash blossoms, I will check inside. For small blossoms, I find that leaving them outside in the shade in an open basket for half an hour or so, and giving them a shake now and then, will usually allow any inadvertently harvested insects to escape. It is best not to wash flowers, but if you must, give them a quick dip in cool water right before using.

Recipe: Party Cheese

As the extravagance of flowers illustrates, the creation of beauty is immensely valuable. Decoration and embellishment are not mere frippery. Gorgeous garlands and arrangements of flowers are considered worthy devotional offerings in many traditional festivals and ceremonies worldwide. It is not only the beauty of the flowers themselves, but the aesthetic effort that went into their arrangement that makes them effective. The simple act of arranging objects into a pattern can be a gift.

For example, suppose you have a block of good cheese and an assortment of edible flowers. Nestle the cheese in a bed of flowers, strew a few on top, and serve it up, and it is a tasty and attractive dish. However, if you carefully and artistically arrange the flowers in patterns over the surface of the cheese, the same ingredients will taste even better, and people may even gasp and take a picture, saying, "It's too pretty to eat." The decorative enhancement adds value, makes it memorable, and arouses appreciation on sight.

This festive dish can be made using any assortment of edible flowers and any type of cheese. If the cheese is hard, it may be coated with a thin layer of softened cream cheese or butter to help the flowers stick to the surface, or use a brick of cream cheese, a cylinder of goat cheese, or a cheese ball as a base. With the cheese at room temperature, use a skewer and/or tweezers to create your flower art, and once decorated, serve the cheese within an hour or two.

Recipe: Candied Flowers

Candied flowers are very painstaking and time consuming to produce, and they add very little in the way of flavor or nutrition. Their glory depends almost entirely on their ethereal frosted effect, delicate colors, and exotic elegance, and because of their beauty and the difficulty of making them, they can transform a humble cottage dish into a royal offering.

Candying is a project—don't try to do it between other activities. Pick a very dry afternoon, as humidity is the enemy of flower candiers. If the day is humid, rainy, or damp, give up. However, when conditions are right, this activity can be a lot of fun for meticulous and artistic people. I have candied flowers blissfully alone with great music, with a beloved elder relative, and in a small giggly group of friends. Interesting thoughts and conversations inevitably arise.

You will need the following:

- flowers
- egg whites
- vodka (optional, but helpful)
- superfine granulated sugar
- small, clean paintbrush and tweezers
- racks covered with parchment or waxed paper

Choose sweet flowers without thick centers, or candy individual petals. If using roses, snip off the bitter white tip where the petal joined the flower. If you don't have superfine sugar, whiz regular granulated sugar in a blender or food processor, or crush with a rolling pin until it is fine but not powdered. Beat an egg white to a soft froth, adding (if available) two to three drops of vodka, which helps it dry.

Carefully paint all the surfaces of each flower and petal with egg white, and sprinkle all over with sugar. Take your time and be a little fussy. When all surfaces are coated, place each flower faceup on a parchment– or waxed paper–covered rack. Place filled racks in a cool, dry, dim, and airy spot, or in a room with a dehumidifier. When completely dry, the flowers will be stiff and very brittle. Gently double layer them in a shallow freezer container with parchment or waxed paper between the layers. Double wrap the container and store in the freezer for up to one year. They may be stored airtight at room temperature for a month or two, but if dampness or humidity reaches them, they will turn to goo.

Of course, candied flowers are spectacular on sweet dishes like cakes and fancy cookies, or on puddings and pies. They can also be used to ornament savory canapes and small dishes, especially those that might be visually bland. If you have broken bits, don't throw them out—they still hold beauty. Mix them into the sugar bowl or sprinkle them over whipped cream.

Other pretty and delicate things, like mint leaves or berries, may be candied similarly, but flowers are the most difficult and provide the pinnacle of this decorative and edible art form.

Recipe: Fritters

I make fritters of all kinds by adding foraged ingredients and/or chopped leftovers to pancake mix, or to an unleavened batter made with eggs, water, and flour (gluten-free flour works best here, but wheat flour is good, also). It gets fried by the spoonful in plenty of butter or in some flavorful oil like sunflower or peanut. If made to impress, they will be small and even; if I'm rushed for time, I make them larger. Eat the fritters immediately or keep them warm in the oven until they are all cooked. Serve with a dipping sauce of your choice for a savory snack, or with honey or maple syrup for a sweet treat. This is a very adaptable recipe—use what you have. Here's one of our favorite versions:

Recipe: Dandelion Fritters

- 3 eggs, beaten
- ¼ cup of water (add a tablespoon or two more if the batter gets too thick)
- ¼ cup of gluten-free flour (a blend with lots of cornstarch)—a bit more if needed to thicken
- 1 cup of loosely packed dandelion buds, whole flowers, OR ½ cup of dandelion petals

Mix batter, add flowers, and drop by the spoonful into sizzling oil or butter. Fry over medium-high heat until browned on both sides.

Recipe: Natural Food Coloring

Edible flower petal juice, from bright orange calendulas to yellow goldenrod to blue chicory, for example, or juice from colorful fruits like strawberries or mulberries, or juice from leaves like red amaranths and dark green nettles, can provide concentrated natural food colorings that can be used to enhance teas and juices, along with cake batters and frostings, cheese spreads, smoothies, ices, and more. Crush the plant material; use the paste or squeeze the juice through a bit of clean cloth. Add a small amount of water if necessary. With some materials, red flower petals perhaps, a few drops of vinegar or a tiny pinch of baking soda may dramatically change the color; this makes a good rainy-day science experiment. It may be possible to preserve the coloring agents briefly by making an alcohol extract, or by shade drying and powdering them, or by storing a puree or paste covered in the fridge, but the fresh colors are always brightest and clearest.

These same plant colors can be used to dye eggs and for other forms of nontoxic, temporary art. Most of them are not lasting, however. For example, the purples and reds found in beets, berries, and red-leaved plants are from a class of colors called anthocyanins.

They are beneficial in the diet and are considered strengthening to the immune system, but they are generally not useful for paints or fabric dyes because they are fugitive and fade quickly. Like berry season, or freshly made tea, or the company of friends, these colors are to be enjoyed vividly in the moment.

Beverage: Mixed Flowers Annual Tea Blend

Making this recipe, especially if done yearly, really tunes foragers in to the cycles of bloom happening all around us, indicating where to look later on for fruits, seeds, and roots. Starting in the spring and continuing throughout the growing season, pick your favorite edible flowers that are just opening and on the young side of fresh. Avoid spicy flowers like nasturtiums, onions, garlic mustard, and chives. Dry them quickly in the shade—not too hot, with plenty of air circulation. (The dehydrator on the "air" setting works well, too.) This will help retain as much color and flavor as possible. If you have trouble with the thick centers of larger flowers molding, try another batch with just the picked-off petals. Layer the thoroughly dried flowers into a sealed container stored away from light. After frost, mix the flowers by gently tossing them together in a large bowl, and store them sealed away from heat, air, and light. Use them as a tea on their own, or as a flavorful and pretty addition to any other loose tea. Mixed with black, green, or herbal tea and packed in a pretty container, perhaps accompanied by a nice teacup, a flower harvest can be a component of a lovely gift. Each year's combination will be different, providing a flavorful record of the past growing season and helping us notice seasonal differences and shifts. They do not store well past the first year, so use them up before spring arrives, bringing new flowers to enjoy.

Practice: A Devotional Altar

Because flowers are only lovely when fresh, they need attention and renewal, both from year to year and from day to day. Effort and energy are devoted to flowers by the plants as they bud and bloom, in the repeated visits of pollinators, and by us when we grow and pick them as offerings. Frequent attention is part of what makes altars, devotions, and rituals so powerful and effective. By tending to them regularly and repeatedly, we begin to carve neurological pathways into untrodden mental territory and form new habits of our choice. In magical work, flowers may be used to represent freshness, youth, beginnings, potential, gifts, and hopeful intentions, making them especially suited for assisting in the process of creation and the formation of new patterns.

You may already have traditions of flower offerings and altar making that you can draw upon. If you are new to this practice, follow these directions a time or two, and see if perhaps you are inspired to create your own flower rituals, fresh and open as the flowers themselves. Flowers remind us that life is a gift, time is fleeting, and everything is subject to change. This is part of what makes them so suitable for making beautiful and fragrant offerings, and why their loveliness and the scents that rise from them are traditionally considered pleasing to deities, ancestors, and many kinds of ethereal beings, including our own souls or higher selves, especially when offered in the context of creating fruitful change.

Here's one way to make an altar. Find a picture, object, or symbol that will focus your attention on your chosen subject. Be creative. If you have no photograph, make a little sketch; it doesn't have to be fancy—this is an altar for personal use. Pick for your focus something you want to honor or increase in your life—a quality, the influence of a person, or a goal, for example. Choose a subject that has repercussions beyond yourself so you can share energy. For example, if I am bringing in healing for my aches and pains, I can say, "May everyone who needs this have it," and then my "ask" becomes general as well as personal. Since healing energy is not finite or limited, this increases the power of the request rather than diluting it. The same holds true for honoring ancestors or other forms of devotional appreciation—the power is amplified by including others.

Set up your picture or object somewhere you will see it, by itself or accompanied by other meaningful items, and put a fresh flower (or equivalent) on the altar every day. When you do, think about beauty, and the potential of beginnings, and how flowers mean the fruit is coming, and how necessary pollination is, and similar flowery thoughts, and link them in your imagination with the subject at hand. I recommend choosing a period within which to offer your devotions—usually daily for a moon cycle or month, but weekly, a year and a day, or some other time period may be more appropriate. Ideally, after the set time has passed, you will find that your chosen devotions and themes have integrated into your general way of thinking and no longer require a physical focus. If this is not the case, clean and renew your altar, and your intentions, as often as you wish.

List: Ways to Eat Flowers

- sprinkle on salads
- stuff with cheese or other filling
- decorate a cheese ball, bar, log, or cake
- add to quick breads, muffins, and fritters
- combine with your favorite dips
- dry for adding to winter teas
- infuse in oil, liquor, vinegar, or syrup

- add to butters, jams, honeys, and sugars
- freeze in ice cubes
- float on hot or cold soups
- flavor butter cookies, cakes, or shortbread
- garnish almost anything

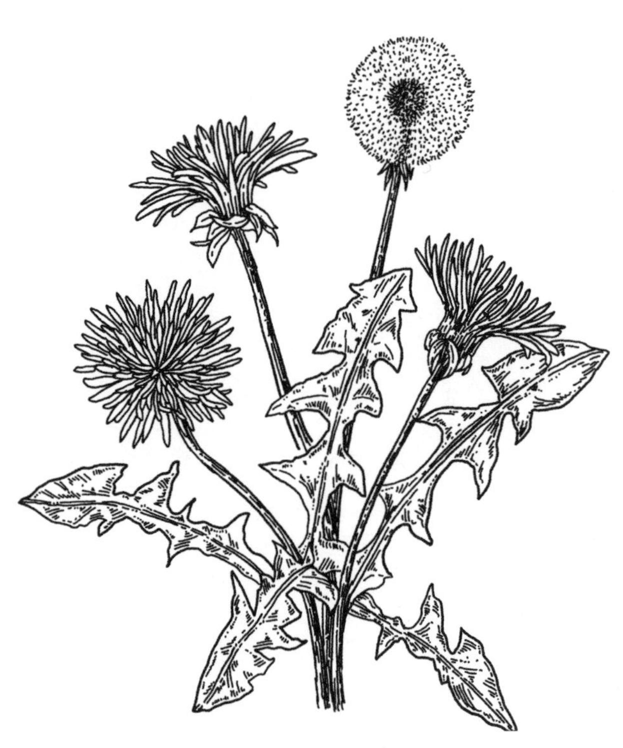

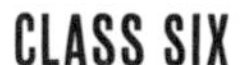

CLASS SIX

Cooking Techniques

Some people date the entry of our species into humanity to the time we began sharing food and storytelling while gathered around a fire. This activity has been nearly universal for most of our history. The people were usually traveling, and for nomadic people, the hearth, rather than the bed, was the defining feature of a home. It provided food, warmth, and protection, and it was the only source of light at night, while at the same time being rather fickle and dangerous.

Building and tending fires is a highly technical art, often with symbolic and ceremonial overtones—explore your own culture for fireside traditions; many of them are very ancient. Meanwhile, be aware that whether or not you can trace your fire keeping heritage, cooking beside a small fire is deep in everyone's roots—experiment with hearthside cooking whenever it is safe and feasible to do so, and you will soon find yourself developing your own personal style, habits, and favorite ways. Building and tending fires with children is an ancient and entertaining practice that also passes on several essential survival skills that a flickering screen cannot provide. Because fires are the original model on which the flickering screens are based, a fire is one of the few things that can lure us to look up. When combined with delicious foraged food, stars, and good storytelling, fires provide a healthy dose of ancient and universal human culture.

The Archaic Kitchen

The wide range of techniques, methods, and materials used for hearthside cooking reflects its long, worldwide history and shows us the roots of all modern culinary arts. It makes good sense for nomadic cooks to forage cookware and kitchen equipment rather than carry them from camp to camp, and to burn rather than wash the dishes after meals so as not to attract predators (like wolves), vermin (like rats), or pests (like ants and flies). Foraging practices include not only foods but the kitchen and its tools as well. Traditional cooking techniques range from the simple and obvious to the elaborate and highly skilled—I will only brush by a few examples here.

WOOD

The wood or other fuel used in cooking can influence the intensity and duration of heat and may provide flavorful smoke. Do not, of course, use any toxic wood—around here, that means making sure no bits of poison ivy are concealed in the firewood. Oleander, rhododendron, and yew are also to be avoided. Some woods, like green (fresh) evergreens and oaks, while not toxic, may add tarry or "off" flavors—use them to start the fire if necessary, then switch to cooking wood.

Many kinds of wood and bark contribute wonderful flavors. The stage of cooking makes a difference—often a handful or two of "smoke wood" twigs are added toward the end of grilling, toasting over coals, or using any method of cooking that allows the food to be bathed in smoke, even briefly. Of course, longer smoking methods, such as those used for fish, bacon and hams, or whole raw eggs, also benefit from flavorful smokes: hickory and apple are particularly favored. Also try the delicious smokes that come from fruit and nut trees, berry bushes, and grapevines. Skillful pruning usually benefits these plants, whether wild or cultivated, and the prunings can be saved for smoke wood. (Make sure if you are using cultivated wood that it has not been sprayed with anything toxic.)

Fresh (green) straight twigs and plant stems can be used as taste-enhancing skewers, toothpicks, and utensils. Children roasting marshmallows quickly find out the advantages of using green rather than dry wood for cooking equipment. Many arrangements of spits, skewers, racks, planks, and branches have been used to hold food next to the fire, and each method produces characteristic textures and flavors. For example, the Native American nations in the rainy Pacific Northwest have a delicious tradition of roasting salmon on a damp cedar plank. This recipe—which uses fish, wood, and a method that are all rooted in the region and its people—has been admiringly translated in restaurants and home kitchens in many places. It makes me wonder what combinations of wood, weather, and local produce might become a world-famous specialty of *your* region?

LEAVES

Leaves, of course, are often food in themselves. Stuffed grape leaves, for example, are eaten along with the filling they enclose, adding flavor as well as containment. But even leaves that are too large, tough, and bitter to be eaten may provide deliciousness and protection when used as a cooking aid like parchment paper, as a dish or platter, or to store and reheat leftovers. I usually use dock leaves for these purposes. Smaller leaves, pine needles, grasses, fungi, and barks can form a nest in which food can be roasted, steamed, braised, or simmered. This method is especially good for delicate items like trout, small game, or fruits. When all the ingredients are collected at the same time and in the same area, the depth and complexity of the synergistic flavors (and nutrients) are unique to each experience.

STONES

Stones hold and disperse heat and have many uses in hearthside cooking. Small- to medium-sized stones can be heated and carefully placed into the cavities of fish, game, squash, and so on to roast them from within. They can be used to heat liquids in containers that could not be put directly on the fire—gourds, for instance, which were cultivated as containers long before the invention of pottery. Submerge heated stones in the liquid, replacing them as they cool. Usually, they are manipulated with wooden tongs or holders made on the spot. Large flat stones may be used as bakestones or griddles. Recipes such as pancakes, biscuits, scones, and pones all have their origins on the bakestone. It is said that in Wales, being so oppressed and poverty-stricken, the people didn't get cookstoves until three hundred years later than the English, and that is why so many traditional Welsh dishes are cooked on the griddle or bakestone.

I must add a caution here. Some people are led to think of stones as inert, but they are not, especially in the presence of water and fire. Some stones may explode, crack, or leave fragments in the food.

How to choose good stones for the hearth is a localized art—try to learn from someone in your area. If you must wing it on your own, here are a few tips. Ask permission and offer thanks, as when harvesting. Use solid and heavy nonporous, non-sedimentary rocks. Let the rocks warm slowly and don't get them too hot the first few times. Rocks that have been part of a firepit are already tempered and ready to use. When you leave camp for the last time, leave the stones a little gift ... like tipping one's server, this is technically optional, but it should be your normal practice, especially if you want to become a regular.

DIRT

Fire heats the soil around and beneath it, while earth absorbs and disperses the heat and energy of the fire. These somewhat opposite qualities can be used to advantage in cooking. There are lots of methods that involve heating soil and rocks by burning a big fire and then using the stored heat for a long bake.

On a small scale, packets of food wrapped in leaves, along with eggs, potatoes or other root vegetables, apples, and so on may be buried in the sand around a fire. Tucked into the ashes as the evening fire dies down, they will be ready for breakfast and safe from being nibbled. Don't neglect to mark exactly where you buried them. To pit roast anything, dig a hole and burn a fire in it. How big a hole, how big a fire, and how long to burn it depends on how long it needs to stay hot. When the surrounding soil is hot and there is a nice bed of coals, place your food on the coals (usually but not always wrapped or contained somehow to protect from grit) and bury everything with hot dirt or sand. The heat will be held in, and without oxygen, the food can't burn, nor can it dry out. Up to about a two-hundred-pound animal may be pit roasted this way, and in that case, it would stay in the ground for twelve hours. Pit roasting is a traditional Native American way to cook beans and was adapted into the famous Saturday night bean pot suppers of early New England. Another Native American traditional method, the clambake, uses a fire-heated pit at the beach, lined and covered with seaweed.

With pit roasting, you need experience to tell when it is done, how much wood to burn, and so forth. Start small and build up your knowledge bit by bit. If your bean pot comes up crunchy, set it over the fire, add water, and turn it into soup. If your pit-roasted food is not all the way done, cut it up and finish it on the grill. Next time you will know better! The terrific thing about pit roasting, when you have figured out the timing, is that once the food is buried, it requires no tending. You can't stir it, poke it, or check it. The fire can't get out of control. All is quiet, cool, and dark above ground. You can sleep, take a hike, go out in a boat, or go to town. You could even get married. When you are ready to eat, dig up your buried treasure and let the feasting begin!

Stuffed Grape Leaves Three Ways

Start looking for grape leaves in June; at first, tender, young, light green leaves will be everywhere. Later in the season, you may need to seek out the growing ends of the grapevines to find young leaves. Any wild or domestic grapevine will do, as long as it has not been sprayed with anything toxic. It's good to take note of any wild grapevines in your area anyway in case you want to check for fruit later. Also, in an emergency, cutting a grapevine and bending it over into an empty bottle will provide you with naturally filtered water in the form of grape sap.

RECIPE TECHNIQUE: TO PREPARE GRAPE LEAVES FOR STUFFING

Pick tender young leaves. Leave the stems on. Wash if necessary. To blanch, use the stems as "handles," or, if you have not left the stems on, use tongs to dip three to six leaves at a time into boiling water, swish once, remove, and drain. They should soften some and turn olive green, but not cook. Continue until you have blanched all the leaves. Trim off the stems with scissors. The grape leaves are now ready to stuff. Or, roll the blanched, stemless leaves into loose cigars, pack into a jar, cover with brine, label, and store in the fridge for up to a year. Or, roll into bundles, wrap tightly, label, and freeze.

Recipe: Middle Eastern-Style Stuffed Grape Leaves

In this version, the grape leaves are stuffed with a filling of cooked rice, tossed with chopped fresh greens and herbs and some good olive oil, and baked.

Optional traditional additions:

- fried chopped onion
- cooked ground lamb, mutton, or goat
- crumbled feta or other sheep cheese
- grated lemon peel

The following version is a Camp favorite: it's a great dish for potlucks and picnics, since it can be made ahead, doesn't spill, and can be eaten without utensils either hot or cold. Best of all, it's on most people's diets: sugarless, vegan, gluten free, and classic.

- 3 dozen grape leaves, blanched (may be fresh, brined, or frozen and thawed)
- 4 cups of rice, cooked, warm or cold (if the rice seems very dry, add ¼ to ½ cup of water to the pan right before baking—any kind of rice will do, but we prefer brown basmati)

- 1 cup or more of finely chopped herbs (such as plantain, lots of lemony sorrel, lamb's quarters, and pigweed—toss with the rice to form the filling)
- ½ cup of olive oil

This amount fits into a large glass baking pan. I bake it at 350 degrees Fahrenheit for about forty-five minutes.

To stuff:

With a blanched leaf facedown on a flat surface, place a small amount of filling above where the stem was—fold up the bottom two lobes, fold in the sides, and roll toward the tip of the leaf to form a finger-shaped cylinder. Generously olive oil a baking pan and nestle your rolls tightly side by side in a single layer. Drizzle with more olive oil and bake in a moderate oven or over low coals until sizzling through and through. Store in the fridge when cooled. These are delicious hot, or chilled on a summer afternoon, but traditionally they are served at room temperature.

Recipe: Vietnamese-Style Stuffed Grape Leaves

This is an excellent dish for fireside cooking. Grilling really brings out the lemony flavor of the grape leaves. Marinate the filling ingredients for an hour or two or overnight in the fridge. Roll each piece tightly in a grape leaf, and grill over hot coals, turning several times. The grape leaf should have char marks. Serve sizzling hot with dipping sauces of your choice.

Filling:

Little finger-sized pieces of the following:

- tofu (any kind, but frozen or pressed holds together best)
- uncooked poultry or meat of any kind
- fish, especially firm-fleshed
- shellfish, including shrimp, clams, and more (I first had this dish with strips of lobster-tail, and it was memorable)

Marinade base:

- 1 part soy sauce or tamari
- 1 part water
- 1 part vinegar
- hot sauce to taste
- chopped garlic and ginger to taste

Optional traditional marinade additions:

- a splash of sherry or sake
- chopped chilis, shallots, lemongrass
- fish sauce

- sugar
- lime juice and peel
- sesame oil

Before marinating the filling, set aside some of this mixture. Use as is, or add green onions, peanut butter, and more hot sauce for an excellent dipping sauce to go with the grilled rolls.

Here's an example of a sauce mixed up to serve with a dozen grilled rolls. Prepare twelve fresh grape leaves by washing and blanching them. Marinate twelve finger-sized pieces of the filling of your choice in half of the following mixture:

- ¼ cup of tamari
- ¼ cup of water
- ¼ cup of rice vinegar
- 1 tablespoon of medium hot sauce
- 1 large clove of garlic, chopped
- A similar amount of peeled fresh ginger root, chopped
- ½ teaspoon of fish sauce
- Juice and zest of half a lime
- 1 tablespoon of toasted sesame oil

Half of this gets tossed with the filling ingredients, and the other half forms the base for the dipping sauce, mixed in a fancy bowl with

- 1 tablespoon of chunky peanut butter
- 1 green onion, thinly sliced, sprinkled on top

Recipe: All Island-Style Stuffed Grape Leaves

These arose from a challenge to make something strictly local, and they became a favorite, with lots of variations. Like other versions, they are good finger food and popular at potlucks. This version is stuffed with meatloaf filling, and I usually make them in little square packets rather than rolls, but they are baked similarly to the Middle Eastern style, in a greased pan, touching one another, in a moderate oven or over low coals until the filling is cooked through. This is also good made with cabbage, young dock, or any other large edible leaves.

Meatloaf filling:

- ground venison or other meat
- cranberries, fresh or dried, coarsely chopped
- chopped herbs
- poultry fat, bacon grease, or other available fat

Optional additions, depending on availability:

- an egg or two
- chopped garlic, onion, or leeks
- grated carrot, squash, or other vegetable
- chopped pepper, hot or sweet, to taste
- chopped skinned tomato with most of the juice squeezed out
- seeds like sunflower or pumpkin
- spices like fennel or celery seeds

Here's a recent popular blend, enough to stuff twenty-five fresh, blanched, preserved, or thawed grape leaves:

- 1 pound of ground venison
- ¼ cup of duck fat (and a little more to grease the pan and rub over the top before baking)
- ½ cup of dried cranberries, coarsely chopped
- 1 cup of chopped mix of plantain, parsley, sorrel, pigweed, green onions, and garlic mustard
- tiny amounts of finely chopped rosemary and yarrow—a scant ½ teaspoon total
- 1 tablespoon of fennel seeds
- 1 egg

This was mixed well and made into twenty-five walnut-sized meatballs, which were wrapped in grape leaves and squeezed together to fit in a greased eight-by-eight-inch pan. The top was rubbed with additional duck fat, and it baked at 350 degrees Fahrenheit for about an hour.

Beverage: Raisin Tea

Raisin tea is an old home remedy for constipation, like a mild form of prune juice. It can be made stronger or weaker depending on the quantity of raisins used and is gentle and suitable for small children and elders. Naturally sweet, it's tasty both hot and cold. Wild grapes you have dried and stored are fine for raisin tea, since it won't matter that their skins may be tough and their seeds crunchy. Other dried fruits such as rose hips, bird cherries, apples, apricots, or prunes may also be used, singly or in combination.

Use anywhere from three raisins to a handful per quart of water. Cover with boiling water and steep until just warm. Strain and serve or refrigerate. Good plain or with a little honey and a squeeze of lemon. Repeat as needed.

Practice: Looking for Circles, Spirals, and Nets

Although grapes were propagated very early in human history, the first cultivated crops were the twining vines of gourds, valuable for dishes, containers, tools, and musical instruments as well as for food. Beans, peas, and other protein-rich legumes, along with melons, squashes, cucumbers, yams, and many other important food plant families share the quality of twining and twisting and forming tendrils. Plants that spiral have long been used symbolically in art and thought. Abstract yet orderly, spiral and vine motifs are full of motion and flow.

From a philosophical point of view, when we consider humanity's place in the universe, we once considered ourselves and our home as being naturally at the center of everything, surrounded by a smoothly moving series of concentric spheres. The implication of perfect circles rotating evenly at constant speed is that cycles repeat unchanged; circles are complete. There is a well-defined and manifest center. Monarchs and monotheists tend to like this view. There is nothing that should or can be changed in such a system.

Compare this with our current understanding of ourselves and our planet as moving on a long spiral path through the void alone, constantly flung forward into new space. Cycles repeat, but differently each time, the center is in motion, and we are always progressing, whether we like it or not. Nothing can or should remain the same, and we are always breaking new ground. Besides mapping our planet's physical movements, spirals are often used as metaphors for the spiritual paths of individuals, reaching simultaneously inward and outward.

As the process of decentralizing ourselves from our understanding of the cosmos continues, our perspective is beginning to shift away from the model of a single spiral path moving through space and time toward something like a network, foam, or web of multiple universes that coexist all at once. I believe modern physics supports this more generalized perspective, but my mind is not abstract enough to really understand what the physicists are saying, and their theories are hard to get my teeth into. Plants, fungi, and the close, even embedded study of ecosystems that foraging encourages can teach us how to perceive and participate in multidimensional networks in a practical, straightforward (and edible) manner. Like the webs of roots and mycelia that support the spiraling vines reaching around again toward the ever-shifting central sunlight, the understanding of our interconnectedness can support and feed personal growth in whatever ways are most effective and most needed. Keep an eye out for these systems in nature and culture. Each has its glories, its drawbacks, and its useful attributes.

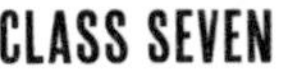

CLASS SEVEN

Working with Fermentation

The term *windfall* comes from the experience of unexpectedly discovering piles of fruit or nuts under a tree after a storm. Finding windfall apples means it's time to make sauce, no matter what else may have been planned for the day.

Usually, when out picking, there will be a specific dish in mind—a salad, or a mess of greens, or a floral garnish—and one can pick an appropriate assortment for that use. Goats work this way, taking a bite of this or that delicacy as they browse, enjoying a wide range of flavors and meeting complex and varying nutritional needs (not to mention finding food everywhere) with their diversified diet.

Alternatively, you may focus on one item to collect: berries, or nettle tops, or clover blossoms. This is the way bees work if they can—the whole hive will harvest one flower at a time, something that is blooming abundantly. Beekeepers often find patches of differently colored, scented, and flavored honeys within one comb of wildflower honey, each patch representing the brief season of a different nectar source. Like the bees, you will usually want to store and preserve your harvests separately.

In any case, there will be times when the intention is for one type of harvest, but then one runs across something else altogether that is especially lush and abundant, that calls out its ripe readiness, that offers itself as a gift of nature. In this case, it's okay to look the gift horse in the mouth and wonder why this windfall has occurred. My mother was fond of quoting her favorite comic, Erma Bombeck: "The grass is always greener over the septic tank."[5] It is a good forager's habit to notice the conditions in which our favorite delicacies grow—history of the land, associated species, slope, water, light, fertility, recent weather conditions, and so on. Such observations can help in finding additional "lucky" windfall harvests in the future. Incidentally, it is also a good forager's habit to carry an extra bag or two … just in case.

---

5. Erma Bombeck, *The Grass Is Always Greener over the Septic Tank* (New York: McGraw-Hill Books, 1976).

Types of Pickling

When you have more than you can easily use or share, thoughts turn to preservation. One especially useful method is pickling. There's a certain amount of confusion and shared terminology concerning pickling that I will try to clear up here. There are three distinct types of preservation:

1. **QUICK PICKLES:** Quick pickles are marinated in an acidic solution, usually vinegar- or citrus-based. As their name implies, they are not intended for long-term storage and are used within three days at room temperature, or three weeks in the fridge. They are covered, but do not need to be sealed. Almost anything can be quick pickled. Small whole onions, hard-boiled eggs, and sliced vegetables are classic candidates for quick pickling.
2. **CANNING:** Pickles that have been canned (usually in jars) have been sterilized and sealed by the canning process. If done correctly, both the organisms that could cause disease and those that are beneficial (probiotics) have been eliminated, resulting in a product that will keep for years and does not need to be refrigerated. Canned pickles, jams, jellies, and so on are great for gifts and for a taste of summer in the dead of winter. It is best to follow a recipe and canning instructions exactly until you understand

the principles of the process thoroughly, as substitutions may be dangerous. It is possible for some kinds of poorly canned foods to look and taste good but be deadly, which has given some people a fear of pickling that should apply only to canning and not to the other types of pickles. This book will not address the specifics of the art of canning, which are readily available elsewhere.

3. **LACTO-FERMENTATION:** These are the classic health-giving pickles of history, found in some form in regions and traditions from around the world. They are made by fermenting vegetables and so on in a salt and water mixture called brine. Fermentation begins at room temperature, and as it proceeds, the pickles change their character, becoming softer and sourer over time. They are not sealed or even covered tightly as gas needs to escape. Once the pickles reach the preferred stage, they are eaten and/or transferred to the fridge, which slows but does not entirely stop the process. Some traditional ferments are aged for years, others are ready in a week or two, and most will keep almost indefinitely in the fridge. If the pickles go bad, it is perfectly obvious—they develop colorful mold, stink, become slimy, and get thrown out. If they look and taste good, they are safe to eat.

Lacto-Fermentation: How-To

If you weren't raised with lacto-fermentation, it takes some getting used to. It's worth it! It is not difficult, and you will not poison yourself by experimenting. Here are the basics:

Food submerged in salt brine naturally develops lacto bacteria; it is their activity that pickles the food, creating lactic acid (sourness) and giving off gasses in the process. Bubbles will spontaneously start to rise after several days at room temperature, then it will bubble vigorously for a few days, then it will settle. The word *ferment* comes from Latin *fervere*, which means to boil or seethe. How long this process takes depends mostly on temperature; the warmer it is, the faster fermentation will take place. When the pickles reach the stage you prefer, move them to a cold spot (the fridge is perfect), where they will keep for years if necessary.

Let's break that down a little:

- **FOOD:** Whole, chopped, or shredded, the range of foods that can be pickled is vast. I recommend starting with vegetables like cabbage and carrots if you are a complete beginner.
- **BRINE:** 2–4 percent brine is a solution of water and salt. Any kind of salt will work, but try to avoid additives; some may add an off flavor. Because some salts are more concentrated, measuring is problematic. You may be precise and weigh your salt to create a

standard brine, or you can use the old method and just taste the brine—it should taste about as salty as seawater or tears.

- **SUBMERGED:** If the food comes in contact with the air, it will mold. Some method must be used to hold the food under the surface of the brine while still allowing bubbles of gas to escape. In other words, air can get out, but not in.

There are innumerable methods for achieving submersion. If you become a production fermenter, you may want to invest in special containers, but for a household, you can use what you have. My favorite fermentation vessels are 1- and 2-quart canning jars, because I like to watch the bubbles working their way to the surface. There are gizmos you can buy, or you can retrofit a brewer airlock—just watch out for clogging when the fermentation gets active. You can use something flexible like a balloon and release the gasses by hand when it gets full—this takes close attention. Refugees ferment in plastic bags that they carry with them, "burping" to release gas as needed.

The three methods with which I have had the most success are as follows.

- Perhaps your container will allow a weight to hold down the solids—sometimes a jelly jar full of brine or a clean smooth stone will fit into the mouth of the fermentation vessel tightly enough to block the food from rising but loosely enough to allow bubbles to pass.

- If the neck of your container narrows slightly, you may wedge (for example) a cabbage leaf and some carrot sticks beneath the surface to prevent floating.
- Easiest of all, a plastic bag or sheet of plastic tucked into the mouth of the vessel and filled with brine will create a flexible barrier that bubbles can push around to escape.

A final tip—if you use ground herbs and spices, they will tend to float to the surface and mold. Whole leaves and spices are easier to restrain. Because of the extractive nature of the fermentation process, they will permeate the brine with their flavor effectively without being chopped or powdered.

Readiness: You can sample the raw food before putting it in the brine, and anytime thereafter. Use chopsticks or a clean utensil, not your fingers, to fish out a piece to try. In the course of the fermentation process, your pickles will go through stages of tasting and smelling a bit harsh, or funky, but it will not hurt to taste them. Once the active, seething stage has passed, the flavors will meld and mellow. As fermentation proceeds, the pickles get softer and sourer. The famous Kosher dill pickles made from whole cucumbers and heads of dill, once sold from wooden barrels on the streets of New York City, come in "half-sour" (still opaque white inside) and "full-sour" (green and semitransparent through and through). The only difference is the length of time spent in fermentation. As another example, some people prefer their sauerkraut, kimchi, or other cabbage pickles to have crunch—others like them soft, or even dissolved into a chunky paste. I might use crunchy "young" kraut as a condiment, while adding soft, sour, juicy kraut to a soup, sauce, or dressing. It's all good—the populations of bacteria vary over time, and so does the flavor, so follow your own taste preferences and form your own opinions.

While all pickles are nutritious and delicious, it is only the third type, fermented pickles, that contains the probiotic organisms that support and repair the digestive system. Just a small sip of pickle juice has settled many a stomach, and it is helpful to those rebuilding their microbiomes following the use of antibiotics or other drugs, gluten intolerance, stress, or any other damage.

Pickle juice—the brine that remains after the pickles have been eaten—has long been known by old wives to be restorative. A dose of pickle juice (from lacto-fermented pickles that have not been canned or cooked) is thought to bring people back to themselves. Pickle juice restores the active probiotic organisms that help promote a healthy digestive system. In doing so, in mysterious ways, it can help restore a person's sense of purpose and intention and strengthen the will. Pickle juice benefits us in many ways to keep our inner ecosystems diverse, healthy, and in balance. When our personal weather gets out of whack, sometimes all it takes to return to a state of harmony is a few sips of pickle juice. We will discuss this more later, but it is pickle juice that points the way.

Plant Portrait: Purslane
(Portulaca oleracea)

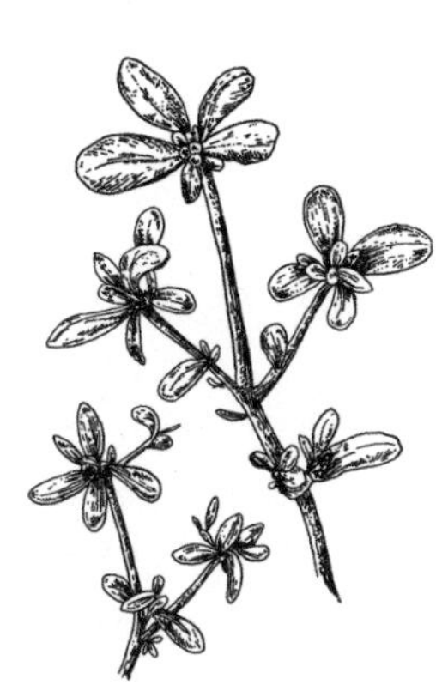

Purslane has names in many ancient languages. It is believed to have been spread around the world by humans as a food plant so early in prehistory that its original home is unknown. It's an extremely nutritious plant, with more vitamin C, vitamin E, and omega 3s than most other greens, and a range of minerals including iron, calcium, and magnesium. It is one of many plants called pig- or hogweed, and it is also called fat hen. These folk names are clues indicating that domestic animals will seek out purslane plants for their nourishing qualities. Purslane is juicy even in dry times and grows very well as a weed in vegetable gardens. Less intrusive than other weeds, it forms low mats so it doesn't shade the main crop, and it can have a beneficial effect as a living mulch, holding in moisture and protecting the soil while its long thin roots penetrate deeply and bring up nutrients. It's quite pretty, with thick, crunchy red stems and small, succulent, green oval leaves. It's usually served raw in salads, cooked like spinach, stir-fried, or added to thicken soups and stews. The texture is somewhat gummy, which some like and some don't. I'm on the edge ... I like the taste very much, but I prefer it in blends or mixtures, dressed with oil and vinegar, or pickled to reduce the gumminess somewhat.

Pickle Recipes

Here are a range of pickling recipes for you to try.

Recipe: Basic Quick Pickles

Mix up a brine by combining vinegar and water, half and half. Any kind of vinegar may be used; each will add its unique flavor, and one may be substituted for any other depending on what you like and what's available. Add any herbs and spices you like—somewhat sparingly, as the flavors tend to become stronger in the pickle. Salt is optional, as is some form of sweetener. Pack the materials to be pickled loosely into a jar and cover with brine. Leave at room temperature and use that day, or refrigerate overnight or longer, up to several weeks.

Recipe: Purslane Quick Pickles

Whole purslane may be quick pickled for an interesting textural contrast—wilted bright green leaves with crunchy reddish stems—but I usually harvest a batch of purslane, strip off the leaves for immediate use in a salad, relish, or soup, and quick pickle the stems for later. Break the stems into lengths to fit your jar, cover with half vinegar and half water, add a pinch of salt if desired, and leave in the fridge until you are ready for a tasty snack or garnish. The purslane has a mild lemony flavor that is delicious all on its own. Because it is quick and mild, it also provides a good base for experimenting with wild herbs and spices. Try a sprig of yarrow or a twig of juniper.

Recipe: Purslane Quick Relish

Mix purslane leaves stripped from the stems, tossed with some shredded spicy mustard greens and/or garlic mustard leaves. Add mustard or other hot or tangy flowers if available. I use about two-thirds purslane to one-third spicy greens, but the proportions are up to you. Add a small splash of vinegar or pickle juice if desired. This mixture is good as is, or with a chopped tomato.

Recipe: Basic Lacto-Fermented Roots

This recipe comes out very differently depending on whether you are pickling chopped garlic mustard roots, Jerusalem artichoke chunks, or burdock root sticks, but the method is the same and the results are all tasty.

- Wash and cut or grate roots into sticks, shreds, slices, or chunks, or leave whole.
- Fill a nonreactive container about ¾ full of prepared roots.
- Add hot pepper, garlic, and whole herbs and spices to taste (optional).
- Submerge in 2–3 percent salt brine, about as salty as seawater or more if you like salty pickles.
- Allow to ferment until active bubbling subsides and the desired sourness is reached.
- Refrigerate and enjoy.

Recipe: Frosty Garden Kimchi

Glean from the remnants of the garden either right before or, if necessary, the morning after the first hard frost. Clean and cut vegetables into pieces of your preferred size—some like large chunks, others prefer shreds; it is strictly a matter of taste. Toss and massage with coarse salt (about one to two tablespoons per gallon of vegetables, depending on the brand of salt) and pack into a fermentation vessel. (I use a glass gallon jar for this.) If your produce is juicy and well massaged, it should produce enough liquid to completely cover the vegetables—if not, add a little water. Keep solids submerged until fermentation subsides and rank flavors mellow, and then refrigerate. Naturally, this recipe comes out differently every year, and I try to make enough to last until the spring greens come in. Garden ingredients might include cabbage, carrots, hot peppers, garlic, ginger, green onions, daikon and other radishes, kale and mustard, celery, and so on. I tend to include wild greens such as lamb's quarters, the stems of mustard and purslane, roots like burdock and evening primrose, and spicy seeds like wild carrot or garlic mustard in the mix. It is perfectly possible to make an all-wild version as well.

Beverage: Pickle Juice Mocktails

Some people in need of a digestive tonic will stand next to the sink, pour a shot of pickle juice, and drink it down. Others devise colorful mocktails and sip them at sunset on the veranda. Children may be tempted by an elaborate presentation as well; especially if you suspect that their upset tummies are related to stress, fixing them something special can be a tangible and effective way to show you care. Pickle juice is salty and sour and often tastes of garlic, spices, and hot peppers, so most mixtures tend toward the savory. Don't add liquor, because you don't want to sterilize the probiotics, and don't add dairy products, which will curdle. Good mixers include fruit and vegetable juices, broths, cold teas, and soda or sparkling water. Pickle juice may also be added to uncooked dishes like salad dressings, dips, and sauces instead of vinegar.

Use the fanciest glass in the cupboard, and make a little production out of it…

- **SOUR MARY:** 1–3 tablespoons of pickle juice, Bloody Mary mix, garnish with pickle spear.
- **GREEN LIGHT:** 1–3 tablespoons of pickle juice, celery juice, sparkling water.
- **SUNSET CRUISE:** Squirt of pomegranate molasses, 1–3 tablespoons of pickle juice, gently fill with carrot juice.

Plant Portrait: Jerusalem Artichoke
(Helianthus tuberosus)

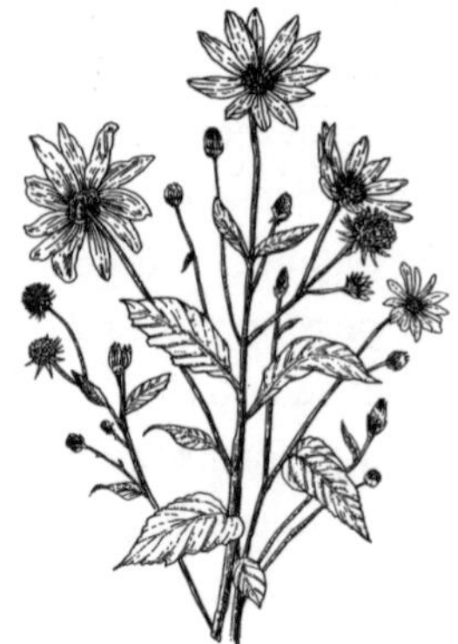

Jerusalem artichokes grow from a starchy tuber, more like a potato than an artichoke. They form dense clumps of tall plants with coarse, rough leaves that bear cheerful bright yellow daisy-type flowers in the fall. They have a reputation of being hard to eradicate once established, but if you ever want to get rid of any, borrow a flock of geese, and they will root up every last shred. The tubers store for long periods and are mild and crunchy, versatile in the kitchen raw or cooked, and especially beneficial in the diets of those with diabetic tendencies. That's because the starch they contain, inulin, doesn't turn into sugars during the digestive process. There's a downside: unless your microbiome is used to them, they can be difficult to break down, causing gas. In fact, some people have nicknamed them "fartichokes." This effect is sometimes reduced or eliminated by lacto-fermentation, which may supply the necessary organisms to help break down the inulin, so Jerusalem artichokes make excellent pickles. In addition to being traditionally fermented, a favorite Southern canning recipe is Jerusalem artichokes put up in a sweet and sour syrup spiced with plenty of hot pepper … although they aren't probiotic like the old-fashioned kind, they are certainly delicious!

Practice: Planting Future Windfalls

Jerusalem artichokes thrive on the boundary between wildness and domestication, and as such, they can help us understand some dramatic differences in cultural perceptions. Actually a North American native perennial wild sunflower, they were cultivated long before colonization, so their ease of growth, mild flavor, and impressive size are the result of centuries of selection for food quality and propagation of the best varieties. They were allowed to naturalize or "go wild" along travel routes, near regular camps, and wherever they could be easily accessed in times of need. Such plantings encouraged the presence of game animals by providing food sources for them as well.

When colonizers came from Europe, their ideas of food production were based on grains and livestock, with horses for transport and oxen for power. This system required firmly established and universally accepted concepts of land ownership and the ownership of animals, physically expressed in boundary walls, hedges, and fences. The word *garden* comes from the same root as the word *yard* (*ardd* in Welsh) and means an enclosed space.

I can tell you from experience that the greatest threat to edible wild plants here on the farm are our own free-ranging flocks and herds of grazing animals and poultry. That's one reason I "forage" in our large fenced and hopefully goat-and-goose-proof gardens and always leave some areas to get weedy, allowing favorites like evening primrose and lamb's quarters to go to seed. Visitors to the gardens typically think these areas are abandoned or neglected, but they are actually being managed for long-term food production.

Similarly, the colonists were not able or willing to see the culture and cultivation that had gone into the unfenced mature food forests of our region. Most of the human cultivators had been taken by the plagues and pestilences that preceded and accompanied the colonists. Credit for the nearly empty, abundant "wilderness" teeming with game and "wild" food of all kinds did not go to those who had developed, cherished, and maintained it. Instead, the bounty of the land was ascribed by the colonizers to the favoritism of their god and to the superiority of their race and culture.

This idea was used to justify conscientious attempts to turn the "savage wilderness" into "New England." For example, a colonial island nation like Britain valued ship building highly, so massive oaks were quickly cut for timber, with no regard for the tons of high-quality food for humans, deer, turkeys, and other wildlife that a single oak tree can produce. Pigs were pastured on oyster beds and on patches of Jerusalem artichokes and other edible roots. Codfish and passenger pigeons were salted down in barrels and sent to the cities of Europe. Dams were built to power mills, and the land was cleared and fenced for pasture. Even the droppings in the bottoms of bat caves were mined and sold as fertilizer to replenish the depleted soils of Europe. In a surprisingly short time, the abundance was consumed or privatized, and only Westward Expansion prevented famine and unrest.

This tragic process continues to play out around the planet as extractive industries that view the earth and its people as resources to be turned into capital come into direct conflict with traditional land use practices that, in general, regard the world and our role in it as sacred. Understanding this dynamic and ongoing history can provide helpful and illuminating guidance as we make choices in our personal lives.

As ethical foragers, we attempt to enhance rather than deplete the places where we live, eat, and harvest, behaving in the woods and wild areas as guests in an ancestral garden. We try not to ruin anything; we try to plant more food than we take, to remove invasives, and to offer tangible thanks to the land and its inhabitants, past and present, human and otherwise. We do this not to make up for the past, or out of any sense of guilt, but to benefit the future, shift destructive patterns, and realign ourselves with reality, as the plants we forage are constantly encouraging us to do. What better way to demonstrate our commitment to an abundant future, and act on our responsibility to improve our surroundings, than to go out and plant some Jerusalem artichokes?

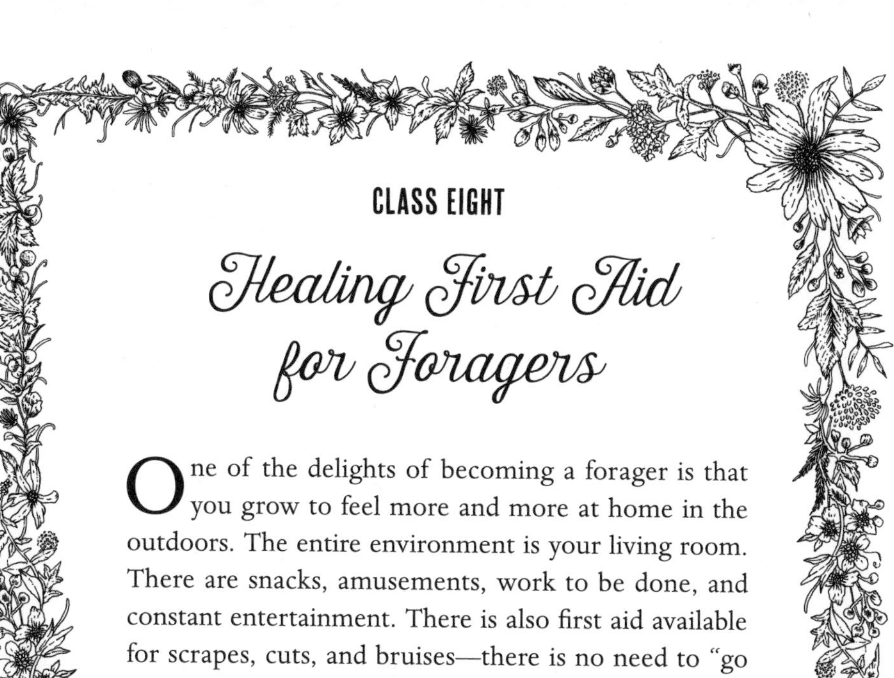

CLASS EIGHT

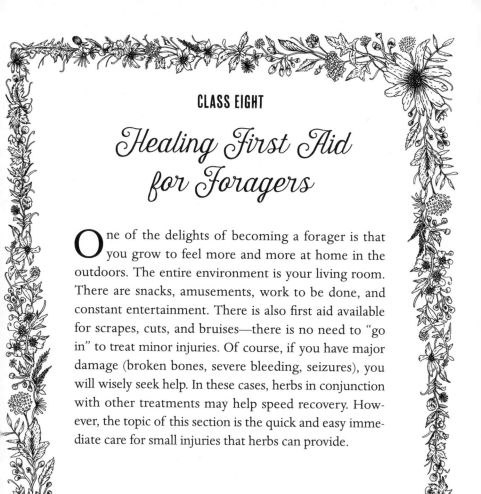

Healing First Aid for Foragers

One of the delights of becoming a forager is that you grow to feel more and more at home in the outdoors. The entire environment is your living room. There are snacks, amusements, work to be done, and constant entertainment. There is also first aid available for scrapes, cuts, and bruises—there is no need to "go in" to treat minor injuries. Of course, if you have major damage (broken bones, severe bleeding, seizures), you will wisely seek help. In these cases, herbs in conjunction with other treatments may help speed recovery. However, the topic of this section is the quick and easy immediate care for small injuries that herbs can provide.

While the injuries we treat may be minor, it is very important to get into the habit of using simple remedies any time the skin is bruised or broken, and also on rashes and insect bites. Many of us who grew up in the age of antibiotics have gotten careless, but this old-fashioned habit has saved many lives. Once infections have taken hold, treatment, whether with antibiotics, herbs, or both, is difficult and outcomes are uncertain. It is far better to avoid infections in the first place by applying a few leaves from one of the healing weeds. Also, the complex compounds in whole plants tend to nourish rather than deplete the immune system, and it is much more difficult for pathogens to develop resistance to them than to refined or "pure" drugs.

Three Powerful Plants for Poulticing

The three herbs discussed here may be used internally and externally; however, their primary use in first aid is as a poultice, which means you mash up the plant and put it on the sore spot. The simplest way, out in the field, is the spit-poultice. Look around and find your plant, declare why you need it (show it the injury), pick an especially nice-looking leaf or two that seem to offer themselves, and say thank you. Chew the leaves. Enjoy the somewhat bitter flavor and the way it brings you fully focused into the present. Appreciate all that the flavor can tell you about the nature and powers of that particular herb—the healing begins right in your mouth. Swallow the juice and spit out the mash to plaster over your injury. If necessary, bind it on temporarily with a strip of cloth or blades of grass. If you can, take a break and let it soak in. Replace the poultice when it gets hot or dry. The spit-poultice is something you do for yourself, and it can be enjoyably used by children.

If you are treating someone else, don't spit on them. Instead, use this slightly more formal method. Put the leaves in a teapot, canning jar, or other suitable container, and pour boiling water over them. After steeping for a few minutes, fish out the warm, wet, softened leaves and cover the injury with them. Sweeten the remaining tea if desired (preferably with honey for its healing properties) and drink some together.

These three herbs are very powerful and very common. Many more "wound herbs" and other medicinal plants are to be found among the weeds and make a fascinating study. However, for the purposes of first aid, these three are usually enough. Each has its specialties, but any one of them, poulticed on an injury, rash, sting, or bite will help prevent infection and promote healing.

Plant Portrait: Plantain
(Plantago major and minor)

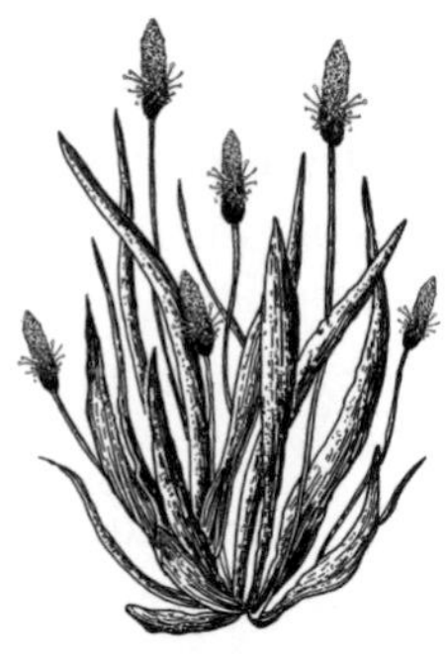

This common weed comes from Europe and was once called white man's foot because it sprung up wherever settlers had traveled. It can now be found almost everywhere. Plantain comes in both broad-leaved and narrow-leaved forms, which can be used in the same ways. It grows in clumps or rosettes, with all the leaves radiating out from the center. The roots form a shallow branching cluster without a distinct taproot and smell a bit like bananas. During the summer, it sends up seedstalks, which also have two distinct forms: in the broad-leaved type, the seeds form in columns up the stalk; the narrow-leaved form has seeds growing in a head-shaped bunch at the top of the stem. Able to thrive under a range of difficult conditions—from mown lawns and gravelly banks to a crack in the sidewalk—if there are weeds around, plantain is probably among them.

A distinctive feature of plantain is the stringlike veins that run parallel down the length of each leaf. If you slowly pull a leaf apart, the strings will be exposed in a way unique to plantain. This is fun to play with. There are several children's games involving the round form of the seed heads. In one, two players pick three stalks of plantain each and alternate taking a whack across the "neck" of the other player's stalk, held out steady, until one of them is "beheaded." (It isn't always the one being whacked.) As each stalk is beheaded, it is replaced, until only one remains: the winner! Another game requires making a loop out of the stem and tightening it between thumb and forefinger until the seed head goes flying through the air; meanwhile, the player chants, "Momma had a baby, and its HEAD POPPED OFF!" The sweeter and more innocent the child, the more they seem to enjoy these delightfully gruesome plantain games.

Such games indicate that the human relationship with plantain is ancient. It was one of the plants that colonized the new ground that was uncovered when the glaciers retreated after the last ice age. Right around the Northern Hemisphere, paleolithic people who followed the grazing herds came to love and depend upon these early succession, magical, healing food plants. The Saxons, for example, passed down stories of the nine sacred twigs (herbs) used to smite the worm of sickness. Plantain was one of the nine—they called it waybread or travel food. (The others were mugwort, chickweed, bistort, chamomile, nettle, chervil, fennel, and crab apple.)

The seeds of plantain are well worth harvesting. Just run your hand down the stalk, or pick a bunch of stalks and hang them in a paper bag until dry and ripe. Seeds from a close relative, psyllium, are the main ingredient in several commercial preparations that add fiber to the diet. Plantain seeds are just as good. Add them to food as you would other seeds, and make sure to drink plenty of water. Alternatively, soak them overnight and consume them already hydrated. Like chia, flax, and other fiber-rich seeds, they can be mixed with liquid and flavorings and left overnight to jell into a healthful breakfast pudding. As a poultice or in an infused oil, plantain leaves are supreme for fighting an itch. From diaper rash to crone's itch after menopause, plantain will bring soothing relief. An exception—don't put oil-based medicine on a poison ivy rash, since the irritant in poison ivy is an oil. A water-based plantain poultice would be okay, but the best plant to put on poison ivy (as well as poison oak and poison sumac) is jewelweed, which neutralizes the irritant, urushiol. Plantain covers all other itches and is also terrific at preventing infections. This is the plant I first learned to spit-poultice—my grandma called it the Band-Aid plant, and no injury I have treated with it has ever become infected.

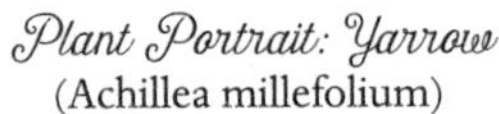

(Achillea millefolium)

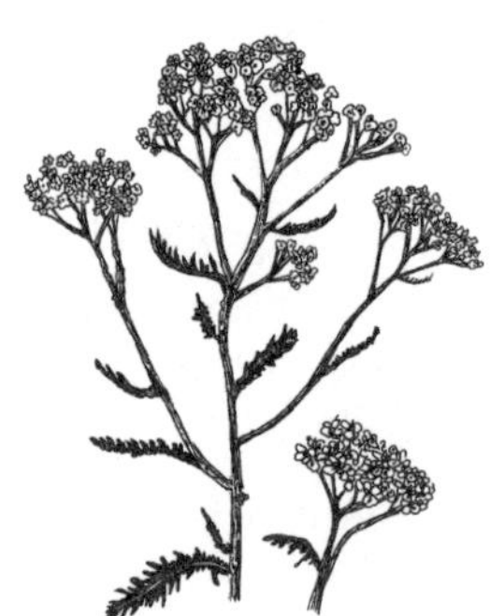

The Latin name *Achillea* is a clue to yarrow's power. This feathery, bitter, common herb with flat-topped white flower clusters is named for a great warrior in ancient Greece, Achilles. His success was due to his prowess, and also to the favor of the deities, especially his goddess mother Thetis, who showed him this herb. With it, he was able to heal his fighters and get them back on the battlefield while his opponents sickened and died of infected wounds. Yarrow prevents infection and is also styptic, meaning it stops bleeding, both internally and externally. Its bitter, sagelike taste is almost metallic, and its use is indicated whenever sharp tools or weapons draw blood.

Found in flower gardens as well as in fields and on roadsides, cultivated yarrows have been bred in different pastel colors such as yellow, pink, and orange in addition to the wild white kind. In general, it is preferable to use the original wild or species variety of a plant for medicine. In the breeding process that led to new colors or growth habits, the medicinal qualities may or may not have been preserved. In the case of colored yarrow, however, the taste and smell seem to indicate that it retains its medicinal powers, and I know of several practitioners who use the colors according to their personal associations, such as pink for matters of the heart, or yellow and orange to invoke solar energies.

Yarrow's strong, tangy, somewhat bitter flavor keeps it from being a potherb or main food source, but its similarity in smell and flavor to garden sage indicates its potential as a culinary seasoning herb. It's great in small amounts in dips, stuffings, and dressings. It pairs well with chicken, game, or fish. As a food or in tea, it has the additional benefit of helping heal internal ruptures, such as ulcers, damage from celiac disease, or any type of internal damage. A further medicinal use is also indicated by its clean, sagelike smell. Yarrow is one of many herbs burned to clear the air in the sickroom, after a quarrel, or on the battlefield.

Plant Portrait: Comfrey

(Symphytum officinale)

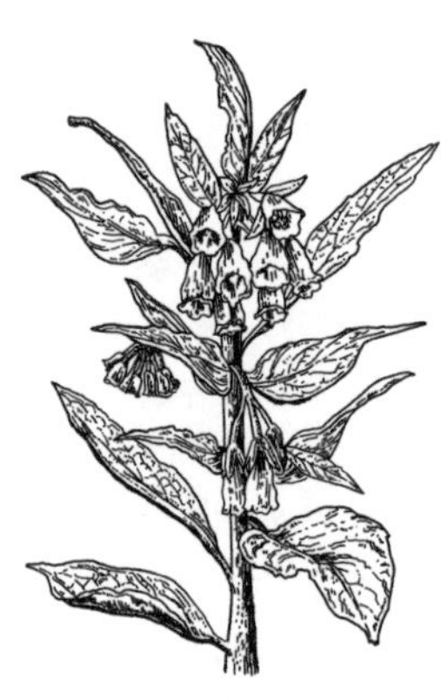

You may or may not have comfrey nearby, but if you do, it is a powerful healer. Be careful where you plant this valuable weed. Once planted, it is hard to get rid of, and trying to dig it up will only make it spread. Never under any conditions attempt to rototill it unless you want a large and very dense patch. The only way I know of to get rid of it is to park a chicken pen over it for a couple of years. Hens and other poultry crave comfrey leaves, which strengthen their eggshells.

Comfrey's folk names include heal-all, hunger bread, and knitbone. The first is partly attributable to the way a comfrey poultice brings increased circulation to an area, helping minimize bruising and allowing the immune system to clean up the injury. It is not recommended to use comfrey poultices on deep puncture wounds, because it will cause rapid healing at the surface, and it is better for deep wounds to heal from the inside out. Hunger bread refers to comfrey's use as food for humans and livestock during famines. Knitbone indicates the bioavailability of calcium and other minerals that can noticeably speed up the repair of serious damage to the body. Comfrey is not recommended for long-term internal use, especially for those with a compromised liver, but I use it internally when I feel the need for calcium, or when I sprain something, and I would definitely drink plenty of comfrey tea and use comfrey poultices if I broke a bone or pulled a tendon. I offer one further caution concerning comfrey—poisonous foxglove leaves have been mistaken for comfrey with tragic results. Since it comes up in the same place every year, get to know the nearest comfrey plant for some of the most powerful healing energy around.

Comfrey is also beloved by organic gardeners as a source of available nutrients for plants. Its large, abundant leaves may be used by themselves as mulch, but usually they are used for garden "tea." By putting fresh or dried comfrey leaves in a barrel of water until they begin to ferment, a powerful fertilizer and immune booster is created, providing great first aid for plants of many kinds, from gardens to houseplants and from orchard trees to bonsai. The "tea" can be strained off and used to water the soil or spray on the leaves of plants that need nourishment and support. The results can be dramatic, since the range of minerals is both balanced and complete. This method of making "tea" for the garden may also be used with other plants, such as nettles, and with manure; in every case, some comfrey in the mix can help activate and enrich the brew. Comfrey does not need to be strained, but if using other plants or manure, be sure to strain out any seeds. The lack of seeds is a big benefit of this method over the direct application of compost.

First Aid Recipes

In summer, when our class took place, there were lots of "wound herbs" growing around us. We could quickly pick a few quarts of plantain, and easily find a stand of jewelweed or yarrow. Fresh plants that you can harvest from, talk to, and leave gifts for, right where they grow, are always preferred when they are available. For traveling or for treating small injuries in winter, however, it's necessary to preserve the fresh plant's healing powers, typically through extraction in oil or alcohol. Here are some basic formulas to call our herbal allies to our assistance at any time of year.

The following three recipes provide treatment for rashes, scrapes, and itchiness. I have never had an oil extraction go moldy, but if it happens, it needs to be tossed, and indicates that there was too much moisture in the plant material. Next time, either use less herbs or allow them to wilt before covering them with oil. I use olive oil, but sweet almond oil and coconut oil are also popular, and in times gone by, animal fats such as goose grease were often used. If you experiment with using animal fats, they should be stored in the fridge or made as needed to avoid rancidity.

Recipe: Plantain Oil

Fill a jar loosely with whole plantain leaves. Cover with oil, label, and store in a cool dark place for a minimum of one month, or up to several years. It may be used as is, or as a base for an ointment or balm.

Recipe: Plantain Ointment

Slowly warm strained plantain oil in a container set in hot water. Add grated beeswax—more for harder ointment, less for soft. Test by dripping it onto a chilled glass or china dish. You will need about an ounce of beeswax for a cup of herb-infused oil. Be patient and careful—the minimal amount of heat is best for retaining the volatile components of the medicine, and wax and oil are very flammable. Pour while still hot into small jars or other containers, and cool completely before putting on the lids.

Recipe: Herbal Balm

Steep a blend of plant materials in a jar of oil, or combine individual healing oils to create a blend. Strain, warm and add wax, and pour into containers as described for ointment. If available, a lump of shea butter and a squirt of vitamin E oil may be added. Classic balm ingredients include plantain, yarrow, calendula petals, rose, St. John's wort, poplar buds, and red clover.

LINIMENTS

A liniment is an alcohol extraction that is used externally. I was taught to make the following two with rubbing alcohol (which is toxic) because it is cheaper and your roommates won't drink it. Also, if you are an overtired field hand living in the woods, they are easy to make and use—pour off the alcohol, stuff the bottle with plants, return the alcohol (with a little left over to rinse out the old bottle), and steep for one month. For a super strong double extraction, the liquid can be poured off onto fresh plant material, topped off as necessary, and allowed to steep another month. The plant material can be left in, and the potion used right from the bottle.

Nowadays I often work with animals and children, so I use a similar process of extraction with an edible alcohol such as vodka. If you can obtain a higher proof form of alcohol, you may be able to make an even more concentrated extract, but vodka works well. When ready to use, mixing the potion with water and allowing it to stand open to the air for fifteen minutes allows most of the alcohol to evaporate so that it is safe to use on subjects who might lick themselves or sneak a sip.

Recipe: Jewelweed Liniment for Poison Ivy

Coarsely chop jewelweed plant tops—stems, leaves, and flowers—and fill a container loosely. Cover with alcohol, label clearly, and store in a cool dark place for a minimum of one month. This liniment should be applied straight or only slightly diluted as soon as possible after exposure, since it actually neutralizes the irritating urushiol compounds in the poison ivy. If applied quickly, it reduces the itching dramatically, and it is useful throughout the recovery process. In the field, jewelweed may be easily crushed for a poultice, since it is very juicy. Smear the juice on any exposure to minimize the reaction and help prevent its spread.

Recipe: Yarrow Tick Repellent

Follow the same process using yarrow, double extracted if possible. I sometimes like to add a lemon peel. This extract is mixed with water (about one-fourth extract to three-fourths water) and sprayed on legs, shoes, dogs, and so on before going out in the field. It will keep indefinitely as an extract, but once mixed with water, it should be used within a few days, and/or kept in the fridge.

Intuitive Recipe Formulation: Making Mouthwash

Although I've compared it to a language, the way we communicate with plants is a series of acts of cocreation. There is no dictionary, and each practitioner, even within a traditional format, evolves their own symbol systems and individual understandings. No one can translate, explain, or provide lists of correspondences for anyone else, because each of us lives in a universe of our own creation. However, I have set down a personal example of this way of thinking that illustrates how expanding the fields of perception strengthened and enriched the foraging experience and its results. Far from blurring the focus with unnecessary subjectivity, adding multiple points of mental reference allowed "homing in" on the best of what the place and time and my own traditions had to offer. It went like this…

My beloved sister called and we chatted about her recent dental surgery. We touched on the subject of mouthwash; although we did not grow up using anything except for saltwater rinses in cases of toothache, we agreed that it seemed like a good idea. The salt water of our childhood was out, because my sister was on a low-sodium diet. "Well," she said on the phone, "can't you make some herbal mouthwash?" This was the essential request. To receive magical aid, to activate the response of the universe and our own inner powers, we have to demonstrate need—and we have to ask. The asking can be a whisper, a shout, or a wail—it can be formal, prayerful, swear full, simple, or elaborate, or it can come as a casual remark, like my sister's. There is a moment when time pauses, as if one had heard a chime, and something connects. People who do intuitive work come to recognize what form this connection takes for them—perhaps warmth, or tingling, or just a sense of knowing—and how to follow its lead, like an energy surfer catching a wave. I felt this feeling when my sister asked her question.

Of course, you can make good medicine theoretically (by following a recipe, for example), but to infuse it with true magic, one must trust the sensed, invisible wave to lift and carry both the healer and the healing process in its own powerful and inevitable direction. This happens best when the need is obvious and the request is clearly focused, as it is when we are making medicine for people we love. It's important to include oneself in this category along with the intended recipients, even if the medicine is not for you, since the healing processes we are working with blend and unify energies like a mandala. By adding various specifics of time, place, and persons, myriad choices may be narrowed down to the most effective possibilities available in the present situation.

In this case, I wanted "mouth herbs" in the form of a tincture, able to keep on a shelf for years, ready to be mixed as needed. We must like the taste, and it occurred to me to make a base and experiment with flavors, since my sister and I have different tastes in food.

All ingredients but the "juice"—in this case, gluten-free vodka—should be growing here where I am at the time when I am making it. There was still a list of options longer than what I needed, so I followed my intuition, going out to pick whatever I had dreamed about, what kept recurring in my mind, and those that had popped up during preliminary research or stood out when I was gathering with my basket.

Often, at this stage of the process, new information will suddenly surface; somehow, the answers to questions will "coincidentally" arrive. Why? Have we tapped into some natural algorithm? Was the information always there and we are just noticing it now because of our new focus? Are our prayers being answered? All of the above? At times like this, we can clearly observe and easily explore the ways we cocreate with the universe. As our perception shapes reality and experience, and vice versa, we choose to ask certain questions and ride certain intuited energy waves. On their backs, between the worlds, we dance. Even when we may appear to be sitting still in the garden, the energetic dance continues, and carries us on.

I was alone, in the surprisingly warm interval in the middle of a lovely late fall day. The sun felt good on my face after being bedridden during stormy weather. I admired the cleanliness of everything after days of scouring wind and rain. I could feel how freshly washed and crisp the little leaves and fronds were as I began to pick them and poke them into a small bottle that had once held sauce. The plucking sound reminded me of grazing, and after a quick glance to be sure that the herd I was shepherding had not gotten into trouble, I remembered the first line of my mother's favorite hymn: "Where sheep may safely graze…" It's the only part I know. I murmured this over and over, and added new lines as they came into my head, as the soft buzz of the song in my throat joined the sounds of birds, humming pollinators, breezes, and the pip-pop of my picking. I picked the leaves that stood out, as if a real one had been placed on top of a very good rendition of the rest. I picked a small flower, waiting until the little greenbottle fly had done with it. This pink flowering form of yarrow grew from seed I had planted the first spring after my mother's passing, and it has thrived in the years since. "Where sheep may safely graze…" I included a small flowering sprig of self-heal as a potentiator and moved up the hill to add some of the wild native white flowering yarrow to my bottle. The herd moved with me, munching loudly. We walked in flowers… food and beauty.

Some days don't feel very magical, and the next morning was one of those. There was rain coming, and my joints ached so much that I hadn't slept well, and walking brought pain with each step. But I had a vision for this medicine, and it required a few more herbs for flavor and action. Ignoring distractions, I grabbed a harvest basket and trudged determinedly.

When I got to the garden, I was surprised and pleased to see that a big clump of lemon balm that had gone to seed had resprouted, so that I was able to pick lots of fresh, tender new growth tips, untouched by insects, and washed by recent rains. The scent surrounded me. Lemon balm can be a powerful antidepressant (keeping in mind that there can be several unrelated causes of depression, each calling for different responses). It makes an excellent winter houseplant, providing a refreshing color and a mild, antiviral tea as well as an uplifting scent.

Although the primary purpose of my medicine was mouth healing, I added the hope that it may lift the user's mood. Considering our family history of depression, I wished us strength to face (and, if necessary, bite) any darkness we might encounter, and I reviewed our personal and ancestral history of cooperation, resistance, endurance, survival, and achievement, which brought us to this point. I felt a resurgence of courage. Pain and loss and daunting histories are the lot of mortals, but lemon balm and borage, and obstreperous fennel, green and pungent, brought me, my sister, and all humanity's ancestors bravely into the present moment. A chill fell over the garden with the first spatters of rain. I returned with a fragrant harvest in my basket, a heart full of gratitude, and maybe even a little spring in my step.

A great benefit of alcohol preservation of plant medicines is that the resulting extracts (tinctures) will stay good for years. When travel restrictions prevented me from visiting my sister, I simply left the jars of alcohol and plant material to gather dust in a cool dark cupboard. One afternoon, when the moon was full (an auspicious phase for bringing things to completion), something got cancelled, and a couple of lovely sunlit hours opened up before me. I rounded up some nice little bottles, a strainer, and a small funnel, along with a few extra lidded jars for mixing, and put some music on.

First, each jar was poured off into the strainer, collecting the "juice" and squeezing as much as possible from the plant materials before composting them. Covering the containers when not in use reduced evaporation. With the plant materials removed, the jars of extracts showed their qualities, each glowing a different jewel color on the sunny counter: some clear, others dense and opaque. Plantain (thick, dark brown), yarrow (clear, light yellow), and lemon balm (clear, foxy brown) formed the foundation. Violet (cloudy beige) and some "food coloring" made by tincturing black hollyhock, bachelor's buttons, and red amaranth (bright garnet) were added; this formed the base.

A jar was put aside for future experiments, and the rest divided in thirds. A different flavoring tincture was added to each—one lemon peel (bright yellow), one fennel (dark brown, almost black), and one peppermint (very dark green). In the process, I half filled a small jar with "slops" and overflow from the blending, with some of each flavor in unknown amounts—a unique, unrepeatable "jazz" version that I will enjoy.

All the ingredients used were good for teeth and gums, and none were toxic, except for the alcohol, and we would not be using enough at once to be concerned. I didn't intend to repeat this experiment exactly, preferring to integrate anything learned on this round into future attempts, so there was no point in standardizing or taking precise measurements. Without the necessity to focus the counting brain, the intuition was allowed to layer on additional shades and degrees of meaning that enriched the effective power of the potion well beyond the capabilities of its physical constituents; it added the magic. While the particulars of your own work and the specifics of your own magically enriching layers of meaning will be different than those in this example, some universals hold true. Appreciation of beauty, gratitude for courageous ancestors, thinking kindly about those who may benefit from this healing's use, and sending well wishes to any and all who may need this type of healing strengthen the work. It is this kind of magic that turns nutrients and chemical compounds into food and medicine, able to transform, heal, and nourish on every level.

Beverage: Tea Medicine

Tea has a long and well-deserved reputation as an ally in challenging times. After a shock or a rescue, after an injury or a death has been dealt with, when things are, as much as possible, back in place, it's not advisable to go rushing off immediately. Strength, stamina, and the ability to recover both physically and psychically, so valuable in times of crisis, are enhanced by a brief pause, a few minutes of respite, a few deep breaths, and a cup of tea. Even on an ordinary day, taking a tea break—making time to stop, change modes, and rest and contemplate—is a proven way to stimulate creativity. It promotes healing and allows time for thoughts to settle and for conflicting urges to come into balance. It's like a reset button, allowing mind and body to touch base with each other, and with the time and place in which we find ourselves.

I make tea in a glass canning jar. You may use any food-safe, heat- and waterproof container, even a teapot. If using dried herbs, steep in water that has just come to boil. If brewing tough materials like roots, bark, and fungi, you want to simmer your mixture awhile, as if making soup. For delicate fresh herbs, fruit, and flowers, use water that has not quite boiled, or make sun tea or a cold infusion. Variations in temperature and different lengths of time steeping (before straining off the tea) extract different flavor elements, so experiment until you find your preferences.

Tea is useful medicine externally as well. Infusions made with hot water and plants can be used as soaks, washes, sprays, and steams. Guided by scent, it may be possible to match the plant with the purpose; for example, mint is bracing, sage is drying, mullein softens, and calendula soothes. However, any nontoxic plant can be used effectively.

Breathing fragrant steam with a towel over one's head is a classic home remedy for respiratory distress. Very hot herbal soaks help keep deep cuts and puncture wounds from getting infected. Tea ice cubes are great for soothing insect bites or sunburn, and those made from chamomile are traditionally given to teething babies to gnaw on.

Also, if stranded without access to any plants, see if it's possible to get a cup of tea. Whether black, green, herbal, or decaf, there is a powerful healing plant somewhere in the background, complete with an evocative aroma. After brewing, the tea bag can be squeezed out and used as a small, neatly packaged poultice. Black tea is astringent, so it's especially good for puffiness, swelling, and tired eyes.

Practice: Stretching with Plants

If you are a practitioner of meditation, yoga, or tai chi, or you are a dancer or an athlete, or you have an exercise routine of any kind, I encourage you to practice in the company of plants. Trees are often used as companions for this sort of practice, since they are very upright, strong, and steadying, but I have had great results working with all kinds of plants, even lawn grass, and I particularly like the sassy can-do attitudes of most of the plants we consider weeds. Exploring their sense of rootedness and the way they reach for the stars (especially the sun) is helpful for developing our own sense of balance, integrity, nature connection, and cosmic awareness. If no particular favorite exercise leaps to mind, try this one. Stand facing a plant of any kind. If no plants are available, imagine them. Sense your roots below you under the ground, and the sky above drawing you up. Breathing slowly and deeply, with your motions following the breath in whichever direction feels right at the moment, reach out to the sides as far as you can, expanding and clearing your space, inner and outer. Reach with your arms and hands, keeping them as relaxed as possible, but reach also with your mind's eye, enlarging and enhancing your energy field. Return to center. Breathing again, reach up as high as possible. Following the breath, reach to the front, including the area behind you in your sense of expansion, and on the next breath, stretch down toward the center of the earth, as if your fingers as well as your feet have roots. Finish in a calm, vertical, plantlike stance for a few relaxed and calming breaths. Repeat as desired. This routine might be considered a speedy version of the way plants grow, and they seem to enjoy being included in such energy exercises.

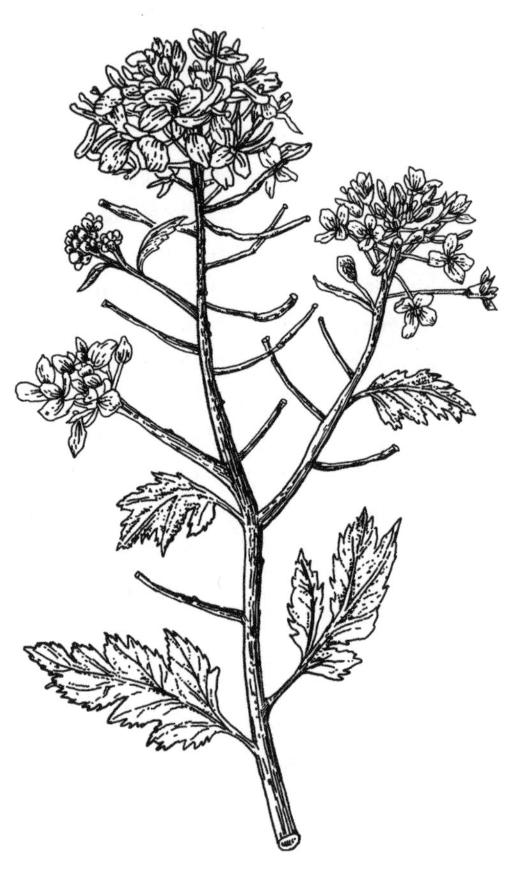

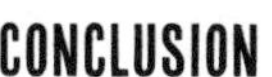

CONCLUSION

Beyond Food and Medicine

The nourishment and assistance plants provide for us extend beyond the physical, emotional, and thoughtful into the intuitive and unseen energetics that we sometimes call magic. One of the things I mean by using the term *magic* is that the ripples and repercussions of these interactions go beyond what we are capable of consciously imagining. While they may remain invisible to us, and be beyond our power to explain, the effects can be profound and compelling, with a reach greater than anything the mind or the emotions can provide. One plant that has demonstrated the magical aspect of nature to me most definitively is stinging nettles, and like magic itself, nettles tend to frighten those who are unfamiliar with them, while intriguing students and lovingly supporting their devotees.

Plant Portrait: Stinging Nettles
(Urtica dioica)

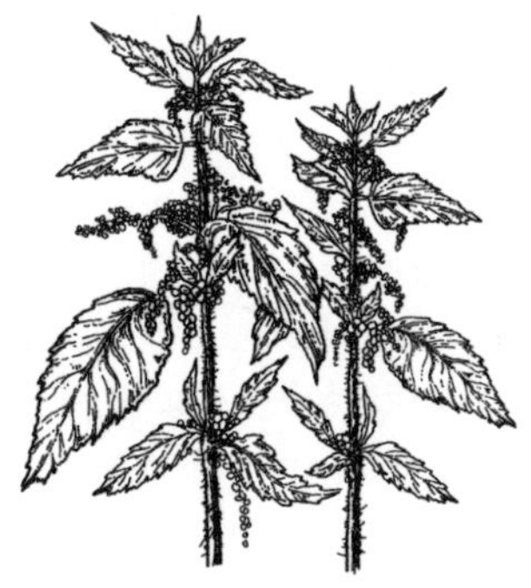

Most people who have encountered stinging nettles by mistake remember every detail of the moment—nettles don't just invite noticing, they assertively demand it. Once having learned the importance of paying attention, nettles prove worthy of notice, indeed. They are one of the most delicious and nutritious of all greens, so rich in minerals that they cause hens to start laying, hair to regrow, and compost to activate. If you like dark leafy greens like spinach or lamb's quarters, simply taste nettles once, and no further urging will be required. Wearing gloves, pick tender tips in the spring and early summer, before the plant begins to flower... after that, the leaves are no longer good for food. Dry your harvest in a paper bag to make winter teas, or rinse them in a colander and cook them until wilted in very little water like any other greens—cooking or drying deactivates the sting—and prepare to feel vigorous.

I feel more vigorous just thinking about a nice dish of nettles or a brothy, nourishing cup of nettle tea. The nettle plant and I are old friends. I have planted and harvested and eaten them, shared them with loved ones and strangers, drunk them as tea and beer, rinsed my hair with them, taught about them, and spun and made cordage with their fibers, which are as strong and beautiful as hemp or flax. I have used the sting medicinally to treat joint pain—what some of my German ancestors called *hexenschuss*, or witch's shot; the helpful effects are similar to those of beestings and last for about six months. Nettle and I have shared many humorous and heartwarming experiences together. I even have a lopsided teacup made by an herbalist and potter, decorated with the shapes of actual nettle leaves, which were pressed into the wet clay before firing.

Imagination is not a substitute for experience, but when based on experience, it can be a powerful force. It doesn't replace the need to go out and actually pick nettles when the season arrives, and I keep a longingly watchful eye on the nettle patch in early spring. However, in times of need, the plants sometimes find another way. For example, when I was sick in the middle of winter and had no dried or frozen nettles nearby, I drank mineral-flavored well water from my special cup and thought vividly about the growing season in the nettle patch and all its stages, and about the roots sleeping even then under the frozen ground. I definitely felt I benefited from magical nettle medicine. Through the use of the imagination, without lying to myself, I was able to harness what some would call the placebo effect for my healing. Although I did not physically consume it, my connection with the nettle plant was activated. Making art, as the potter did, can be another way of exchanging energy with a plant, and there are many documented stories of people in need—prisoners, for example—being visited by healing plants in dreams or visions and experiencing positive mental and physical effects, along with an undeniable strengthening of the spirit.

So … it is not necessary to be in physical relation to a plant in order to use it. Don't be shy about engaging with plants on nonmaterial levels as well as using them for food and healing. Their range of activities can cover all the realms we recognize and more besides, and they know our histories and capabilities better than we do ourselves. A fierce, friendly, and well-defended plant like nettle is a great companion for wandering in timeless imaginal worlds where miracles, revelations, and healing can occur. Their combination of extreme protection and deep nurturance is unique. And when ready to return to the here and now and be fully physically present, nettle can help there, too, whether with a grounding dose of mineral-rich nutrition or a medicinal and attention-getting sting.

Conclusion

Our Invisible Lives

In the beginning of this book, we discussed the oxygen–carbon dioxide exchange continually taking place as we breathe with plants. But this is not the only set of unseen interactions going back and forth between ourselves, the plants, and the rest of the world.

The microbiome, or inner ecosystem, mentioned in the pickle chapter, was once thought to live primarily in the gut. Now, thanks to the ability of scientists to look more closely at our genes, it's been discovered that these interlocking communities of microscopic beings exist not only *in* us and *on* us, they *are* us. Only 10 percent of the cells in the human body (by count) have human DNA. The rest are bacteria, viruses, fungi, and entire extended families of widely assorted forms of life, helping to create, maintain, and break down not only our dense physical bodies, but also dispersing themselves all around us in accompanying clouds of living particles that are part of us, too. This understanding contributes a useful, tangible physical component to working with our personal energy fields or auras, which of course have purely energetic aspects as well.

When sitting with plants, whether silently meditating or in conversation, actively picking or observing from a slight distance, even if we never take a nibble or leave an offering, multiple exchanges are taking place. Plants, animals, people, and landscapes all have characteristic microbiomes, and we and they are always in flux. A close examination of a person's microbiome would show traces of all their exposures and experiences over the course of a lifetime. One reason a plant ally may be especially good for a particular individual is that it specifically supports their unique microbiome's ability to find balance. Foods that do this are called probiotics, because they seed and feed a helpful range of organisms in the digestive system. Some plants, particularly aromatic herbs, perform this helpful cultivation of our microbiome right in the atmosphere. Yarrow, mugwort, sage, cedar or juniper, pine, citrus peel, tulsi basil, thyme, and many more are known for their ability to clear the air, reduce the transmission of disease, and promote healing, by their scent alone or in the form of scented smokes or steams.

Although we are often taught to think of microbes in terms of germs, or disease-causing pathogens, in reality, one of the main things protecting us from dangerously invasive organisms is a rich, dense, and diverse community of in-house organisms—those that are part of us. One of the dangers of broad-spectrum antibiotic use is that our naturally busy, buzzing, fully populated, hardworking native microcommunities get depleted, leaving us open to secondary infections and reoccurrences. Like a neighborhood full of bombed-out buildings, there is room for opportunistic parasites and pathogens to take hold, which don't necessarily have the best interests of the wider community at heart. Our microbiomes can also become depleted through exposure to harsh chemicals, overly processed foods, disease, grief, and stress. One of the best, most efficient, and most delicious ways to restore diversity and healthy resilience to a weakened microbiome is to snack frequently on a wide range of fresh, raw, wild, and/or fermented foods—the more variety, the better. When we nibble and graze while foraging, we partake of food value and nutrition from the plants and places around us, and at the same time, we absorb, take in, and brush against innumerable bacteria, yeasts, and other invisible components of the living world that keep us healthy, balanced, complete, and in touch. When we serve and share our foraged harvests, especially if fresh, raw, or pickled in traditional ways, we help synchronize the microbiomes of ourselves and our companions, and also those of ourselves and the environment that supports and feeds us.

This process of coming into alignment on a microbial level—and through other invisible forms of connection—is part of what makes responsible foraging an excellent tool for connecting with land, and with those who have loved a specific place and eaten and lived there in the past. As we bring our microbiomes into congruence, we may find ourselves sharing thoughts and values as well. Some of what was formerly lumped under relatively vague concepts like intuition or instinct or innate wisdom is now believed to be partly the gut reaction of the highly sensitive and responsive microbiome to the vicissitudes and particularities of life. As elsewhere discussed, the fact that plants are, evolutionarily speaking, much older than animals implies that, in general, their chemistry guides ours, and when we get out of balance, the plants, who created that balance in the first place, may have the power and influence to set us right.

This is another instance in which our view of the world and our place in it is shifting away from a conception of ourselves as lone, independent individuals (or a unique, dominant species). That kind of exceptionalism, along with an "us against the world" mentality, no longer seems to fit the facts. The life and nutrient cycles, the oxygen–carbon dioxide exchange, our intermingling microbiomes, and the ideas we get from breathing together—literally, *inspiration*—all link us to plants and to the rest of nature, as active participants in a web of mutual influence too complex for us to completely comprehend, and certainly far too complex for us to bring under conscious control.

The inputs of numerous life-forms—each with their own perspectives—through intuition and awareness, can bring us wide-ranging wisdom, a depth of happiness, and a knack for survival that the individual conscious mind can never achieve on its own. Our inner ecosystems, in all their diversity, connect us with the world around us, and reveal glimpses of life's multiverse, beyond the reach of our limited perception. And who will guide us in this bustling, blooming, confusing collage of experience? We can breathe easy—we are not breaking new ground here. We know we can count on our committed mentors, teachers, and friends among the common weedy plants to show us the way.

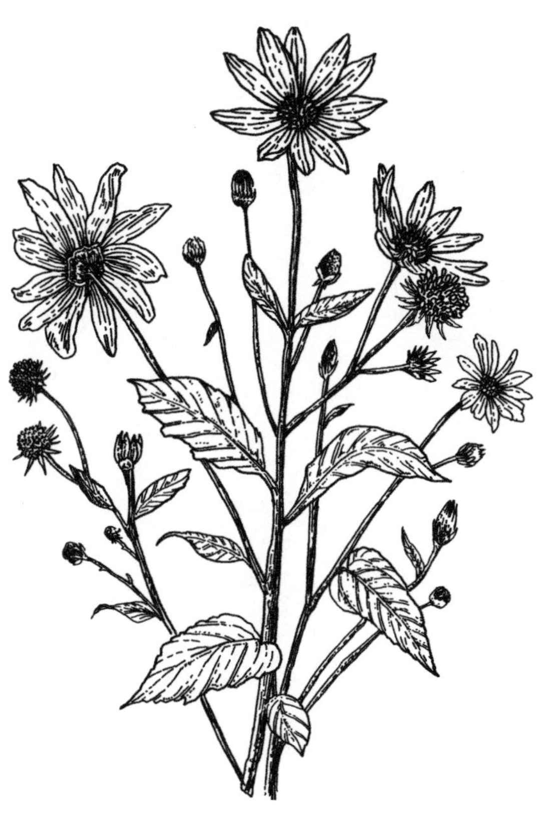

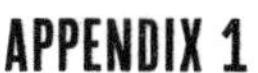

APPENDIX 1

List of Names and Origins

Here is a list of plants mentioned in this book as I have referred to them, usually by the common name with which I am familiar. Since common names vary widely, the Latin name that follows is definitive, since it belongs to only one plant (or plant family). Finally, I have included information about the original range of the plant. This is the region where it comes from and where the most variable, wild, and weedy ancestral forms of the plant may usually be found.

Amaranth	*Amaranthus* spp.	Americas
Anise hyssop	*Agastache foeniculum*	North American Plains
Apple	*Malus domestica*	Central Asia
Arugula	*Eruca vesicaria*	Mediterranean
Autumn olive	*Elaeagnus umbellate*	Asia
Bachelor's buttons	*Centaurea cyanus*	Europe
Barberry	*Berberis* spp.	mostly Europe, Africa, Asia
Basil	*Ocimum basilicum*	Mediterranean
Bayberry	*Myrica gale*	Atlantic Europe, Northern North America
Bean	*Fabaceae* (especially *Phaseolus* spp.)	Americas
Beet	*Beta vulgaris*	Middle East
Bergamot	*Monarda fistula* or *Monarda didyma*	North America
Bittercress	*Barbarea vulgaris, Cardamine bulbosa, Cardamine hirsuta*	worldwide
Bittersweet	*Celastrus orbiculatus*	China

Black locust	*Robinia pseudoacacia*	North America
Blackberry	*Rubus* spp.	worldwide, European is most common here
Blueberry	*Vaccinium* spp.	North America
Borage	*Borago officinalis*	Mediterranean
Burdock	*Arctium lappa* and spp.	Europe and Asia
Cabbage	*Brassica oleracea*	Coastal Europe
Capers	*Capparis spinosa*	Mediterranean
Carnation	*Dianthus caryophyllus*	Mediterranean
Carolina allspice	*Calycanthus floridus*	Southeast North America
Carrot	*Daucus carota*	Europe and Southwest Asia
Catbrier	*Smilax rotundifolia Smilax* spp.	worldwide, twenty species in North America
Catnip	*Nepeta cataria*	Eastern Europe
Cedar	*Juniperus virginiana*	Eastern North America
Celery	*Apium graveolens*	Mediterranean
Chamomile	*Matricaria chamomilla*	Southeast Europe
Chervil, wild	*Anthriscus sylvestris*	Europe

Chestnut	*Castanea* spp. (especially *Castanea dentata*)	Eastern North America
Chia	*Salvia* spp.	Central and Southern Mexico
Chickweed	*Stellaria media*	Eurasia
Chicory	*Cichorium intybus*	Europe
Chives	*Allium schoenoprasum*	Europe, Americas, Asia
Chrysanthemum	*Chrysanthemum indicum*	East Asia, Northeastern Europe
Cinnamon	*Cinnamomum* spp.	Asia and South Pacific
Clover	*Trifolium* spp.	Europe
Coconut	*Cocos nucifera*	the tropics
Coffee	*Coffea* spp.	Africa and tropical Asia
Comfrey	*Symphytum* spp.	Europe
Coriander	*Coriandrum sativum*	Southern Europe, North Africa, South Asia
Corn	*Zea mays*	Southern Mexico
Crab apple	*Malus sylvestris*	temperate Northern Hemisphere

Cranberry	*Vaccinium oxycoccos*	temperate Northern Hemisphere
Cresses	*Barbarea* spp., *Cardamine* spp.	temperate Northern Hemisphere
Crocus	*Crocus* spp.	North Africa, South Central Europe, Asia
Daffodil	*Narcissus* spp.	Southern Europe, North Africa
Dahlia	*Dahlia pinnata*	Mexico and Central America
Daisy (English)	*Bellis perennis*	Europe
Dame's rocket	*Hesperis matronalis*	Mediterranean, Central Asia
Dandelion	*Taraxacum officinale*	Europe
Dayflower	*Commelina communis*	Southeast Asia
Daylily	*Hemerocallis* spp.	Eastern Asia
Dill	*Anethum graveolens*	Europe, Asia, North Africa
Dock	*Rumex crispus* and spp.	Europe and Western Asia
Elder	*Sambucus* spp.	temperate Northern Hemisphere

Elecampane	*Inula helenium*	Europe and North Asia
Evening primrose	*Oenothera* spp.	North, Central, and South America
Fennel	*Foeniculum vulgare*	Mediterranean
Flax	*Linum usitatissimum*	North temperate Europe and Asia
Foxglove	*Digitalis purpurea*	Europe, Western Asia, Northwestern Africa
Garlic	*Allium* spp.	Central Asia, Iran
Garlic mustard	*Alliaria petiolate*	Europe, Western and Central Asia
Geranium	*Geranium* spp.	Mediterranean, temperate regions
Ginger	*Zingiber officinale*	Maritime Southeast Asia
Gladiola	*Gladiolus* spp.	Africa, Asia, Mediterranean
Goldenrod	*Solidago* spp.	primarily North America
Gourd (bottle)	*Lagenaria siceraria*	Southern Africa, from 1300 BC or earlier

Grape	*Vitis* spp.	Middle East
Hibiscus	*Hibiscus* spp.	worldwide, temperate and tropical
Hickory	*Carya* spp.	North America and Asia
Hollyhock	*Alcea* spp.	Asia and Europe
Honeysuckle	*Lonicera japonica*	Eastern Asia
Horehound	*Marrubium vulgare*	Africa, Central Asia, Europe
Horseradish	*Armoracia rusticana*	Southeastern Europe, Western Asia
Hyssop	*Hyssopus officinalis*	Southern Europe, Middle East, Caspian
Jasmine	*Jasminum officianale*	Eurasia, Southern Pacific, Oceania
Jerusalem artichoke	*Helianthus tuberosus*	Central North America
Johnny-jump-up	*Viola tricolor*	Europe
Juniper	*Juniperus communis*	Northern Hemisphere
Kiwi, hardy	*Actinidia arguta*	Eastern Asia, Himalayas
Knotweed	*Fallopia japonica*	East Asia

Kudzu	*Pueraria* spp.	East and Southeast Asia
Lamb's quarters	*Chenopodium* spp.	*berlandieri* (American origin) and *alba* (European)
Lavender	*Lavendula* spp.	Europe, North Africa, Mediterranean
Laverbread	*Porphyra umbilicalis*	West coastal Britain
Leek	*Allium* spp.	Southern Europe, Western Asia
Lemon	*Citrus limon*	South Asia
Lemon balm	*Melissa officianalis*	Europe, Mediterranean, Central Asia
Lemongrass	*Cymbopogon citratus* and spp.	Asia, Africa, Southern Pacific
Lemon myrtle	*Backhousia citriodora*	Australia
Lemon verbena	*Aloysia citrodora*	South America
Lettuce	*Lactuca sativa*	North Africa
Lilac	*Syringa vulgaris*	Southeastern Europe
Lime	*Citrus* x *latifolia* and other hybrids	Southeast Asia
Linden	*Tilia americana* and spp.	temperate Northern Hemisphere

Milkweed (common)	*Asclepias syriaca*	Africa, North and South America
Mint	*Mentha* spp.	temperate worldwide
Mullein	*Verbascum* spp.	Europe, Asia
Multiflora rose	*Rosa multiflora*	Eastern Asia
Mustards	*Sinapis alba* (white) *Sinapis arvensis* (field) *Brassica nigra* (black)	Europe, Africa, Asia
Myrtle	*Vinca minor*	Europe, North Africa, Southwest Asia
Nasturtium	*Tropaeolum majus* and other spp.	South and Central America
Nettle	*Urtica dioica*	Europe, North Africa, Asia
Oak	*Quercus* spp.	Northern Hemisphere
Okra	*Abelmoschus esculentus*	West Africa, Southeast Asia
Oleander	*Nerium oleander*	Mediterranean
Olive	*Olea europaea*	Mediterranean
Onion	*Allium cepa*	Central Asia
Oregano	*Origanum vulgare*	Eurasia, Mediterranean

Oxalis	*Oxalis* spp.	worldwide, except polar
Pansy	*Viola tricolor* var. *hortensis*	Europe, Western Asia
Parsley	*Petroselinum crispum*	Mediterranean
Paw paw	*Asimina triloba*	Eastern North America
Pea	*Pisum sativum*	Southwest Asia, Northeast Africa
Pear	*Pyrus*	Europe, North Africa, Asia
Pennyroyal	*Mentha puligium*	Europe, North Africa, Middle East
Pepper (black)	*Piper nigrum*	South India
Peppergrass	*Lepidium* spp.	worldwide
Peppermint	*Mentha* x *piperita*	Europe, Middle East
Pepperweed	*Lepidium virginicum*	North and Central America
Phragmites	*Phragmites australis*	Europe, Asia
Pine	*Pinus* spp.	Northern Hemisphere
Plantain	*Plantago major* and *minor*	Europe, Northern and Central Asia

Poison ivy	*Toxicodendron radicans*	Asia, Eastern North America
Poison sumac	*Toxicodendron vernix*	Eastern North America
Poke	*Phytolacca americana*	Eastern North America
Potato	*Solanum tuberosum*	Peru
Primrose	*Primula vulgaris*	Europe, North Africa, Southeast Asia
Psyllium	*Plantago* spp.	Europe
Pumpkin	*Cucurbitaceae*	North America
Purslane	*Portulaca oleracea*	worldwide
Radish	*Raphanus sativus*	Asia
Ramps	*Allium tricoccum*	Eastern North America
Raspberry	*Rubus* spp.	Northern Hemisphere
Redroot pigweed	*Amaranthus retroflexus*	tropical America
Rice	*Oryza* spp.	Asia, Africa
Rose	*Rosa* spp.	Asia, Europe, North Africa, North America

Sage	*Salvia officianalis*	Mediterranean
Sarsaparilla	*Smilax* spp.	tropics and subtropics worldwide
Self-heal	*Prunella vulgaris*	entire Northern Hemisphere
Sesame	*Sesamum indicum*	sub-Saharan Africa
Shallot	*Allium cepa*	Central or Southwest Asia
Shepherd's purse	*Capsella bursa-pastorus*	Europe and Anatolia
Snapdragon	*Antirrhynum majus* and spp.	Europe, North America, North Africa
Sorrel	*Rumex acetosa*	Eurasia and Britain
Spearmint	*Mentha spicata*	Europe, Southern Asia
Spruce	*Picea*	Northern temperate regions worldwide
Squash	*Cucurbitaceae*	Andes, Mesoamerica
Sumac	*Rhus typhina* and spp.	temperate regions worldwide
Sunflower	*Helianthus annuus*	North and Central America
Sweet pepperbush	*Clethra alnifolia*	Eastern North America

Tea	*Camellia sinensis*	Southwest China
Thistle	*Cirsium arvense*	Southeast Europe and Asia
Thyme	*Thymus vulgaris* and spp.	North Africa, Western Asia
Tobacco	*Nicotiana tabacum* and spp.	Caribbean, Sub-tropical America
Tomato	*Solanum lycopersicum*	Western South America, Central America
Tulip	*Tulipa*	Southern Europe to Central Asia
Turnip	*Brassica rapa*	Western Asia, Europe
Violet	*Viola odorata*	primarily temperate Northern Hemisphere
Wheat	*Triticum* spp.	Central Asia, Mediterranean
Wineberry	*Rubus phoenicolasius*	China, Japan, Korea
Wintergreen	*Gaultheria procumbens*	North America
Yarrow	*Achillia millefolium*	temperate Northern Hemisphere
Yew	*Taxus baccata*	Europe, North Africa, Iran, Central Asia

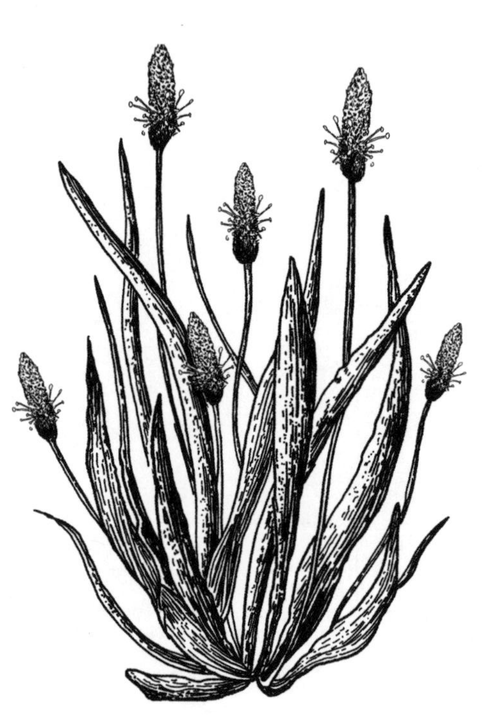

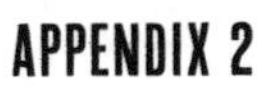

APPENDIX 2

Partial List of Edible Flowers

Anise hyssop
Apple blossom (in moderation)
Arugula
Bachelor's buttons
Basil
Bergamot
Black locust
Blueberry
Borage
Calendula
Carnation
Carrot
Catnip
Chamomile
Chickweed
Chicory
Chrysanthemum
Citrus blossom
Clover (in moderation)
Coriander
Dahlia
Daisy
Dandelion
Dayflower
Daylily
Dill
Elderflower (no stems)

Evening primrose
Fennel
Garlic mustard
Gem marigold
Geranium (scented)
Gladiola
Goldenrod
Hibiscus
Hollyhock
Honeysuckle
Hyssop
Jasmine
Johnny-jump-up
Lavender
Lilac
Linden
Mint
Mullein
Mustard
Myrtle (in moderation)
Nasturtium
Okra
Oregano
Pansy
Pear blossom (in moderation)
Primrose
Radish
Rosemary
Rose
Sage
Snapdragon
Thyme
Tulip
Turnip
Violet
Yarrow

General Index

D

F

G

H

I

J

K

L

M

N

O

P

Q

R

W

Y

To Write to the Author

If you wish to contact the author or would like more information about this book, please write to the author in care of Llewellyn Worldwide Ltd. and we will forward your request. Both the author and the publisher appreciate hearing from you and learning of your enjoyment of this book and how it has helped you. Llewellyn Worldwide Ltd. cannot guarantee that every letter written to the author can be answered, but all will be forwarded. Please write to:

Rebecca Gilbert
℅ Llewellyn Worldwide
2143 Wooddale Drive
Woodbury, MN 55125-2989

Please enclose a self-addressed stamped envelope for reply, or $1.00 to cover costs. If outside the U.S.A., enclose an international postal reply coupon.

Many of Llewellyn's authors have websites with additional information and resources. For more information, please visit our website at http://www.llewellyn.com.

Notes

Notes

Notes

Notes

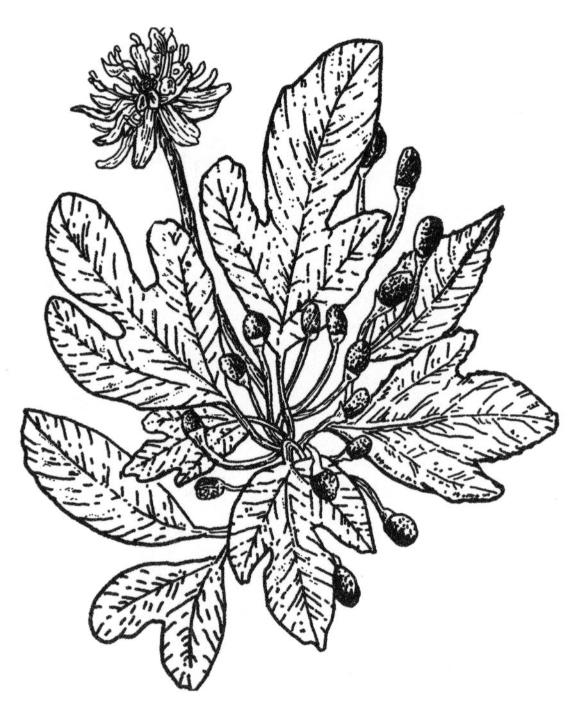